Love Your Cholesterol
The Aging Solution

By Raymond Adamcik, M.D.

ISBN-13: 978-1508587842
ISBN-10: 1508587841

DEDICATION

Dedicated to the advancement of health through knowledge.

CONTENTS

ACKNOWLEDGMENTS

Many thanks to those who were instrumental in the writing of this book. First to my family, Vera, Tyler, Raygen and Ryan, who were supportive of my efforts and who sacrificed their time so that this could come to fruition. I acknowledge the critical information sources that lead me to this junction, specifically A4M – the Ant-aging association of America and Dr. Hurteau, a world leader in anti-aging medicine that inspired me to continue my quest for knowledge.

INTRODUCTION

THE BODY is a miraculous chemical factory. It takes life-giving food nutrients and is able to produce energy. It can grow to amazing size, speed, power and intelligence. It produces, functions, and maintains its advanced brain and neurologic system that is unparalleled in our universe. At the center of all this magic, is the villainized cholesterol molecule. The body is not trying to kill itself. It is performing these functions because they have allowed us to survive at the top of the food chain for 3 million years. It is trying to survive.

WE are trying to kill our bodies! We are poisoning it with life-shortening "foods" that lead to the body's aging and degradation process. We poison it with tobacco, alcohol, medicines, sleep deprivation, and inactivity. Then our bodies are further weakened by hormonal decline. The result is rapid aging, disease, and early death.

You can learn the secrets of a long, healthy and fulfilling life, read on!

Chapter 1

LOW CHOLESTEROL
– IS IT ALL THAT ITS MADE OUT TO BE?

Cholesterol Kills! Eat a Low-fat diet!

Everybody "knows" this. Cholesterol is the stuff that clogs your arteries. It causes heart attacks and strokes. You must lower your cholesterol because you don't want a heart attack or stroke, and everybody wants in on the game. The food industry is a key player in this deception. Labels commonly read "contains no cholesterol". Eat oatmeal to lower your cholesterol", or worse yet "eat honey nut cheerios to lower your cholesterol"! There is not a food on the self that isn't contrived to accomplish this goal. Eat egg whites because the yolk has cholesterol! Mazola corn oil lowers cholesterol!

The pharmaceutical industry is also a player in is deception. Statin medicines were derived for this purpose. In earlier studies, high risk patients benefited from them. The medicine decided that if it was good for a few, let's give them to everybody! Let's wipe out this cholesterol fiend. But is cholesterol really the fiend it is made out to be? Check out this study from the World Health Organization. It is looking at cardiovascular deaths versus total cholesterol levels and BEHOLD! It shows the opposite of what you have been told!

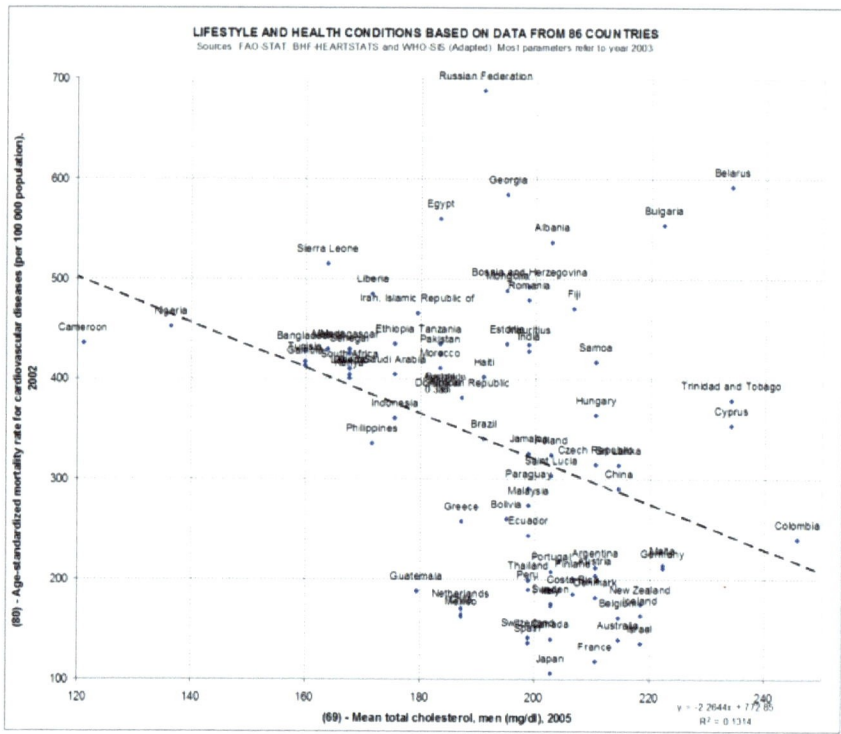

Figure 1-1 THE HIGHER THE CHOLESTEROL, THE LOWER THE CARDIOVASCULAR RISK!

Yet the fight against this "evil" wages on in full swing.

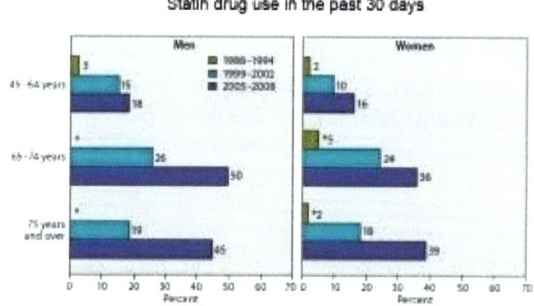

Figure 1-2 – Explosion of statin prescriptions to lower cholesterol

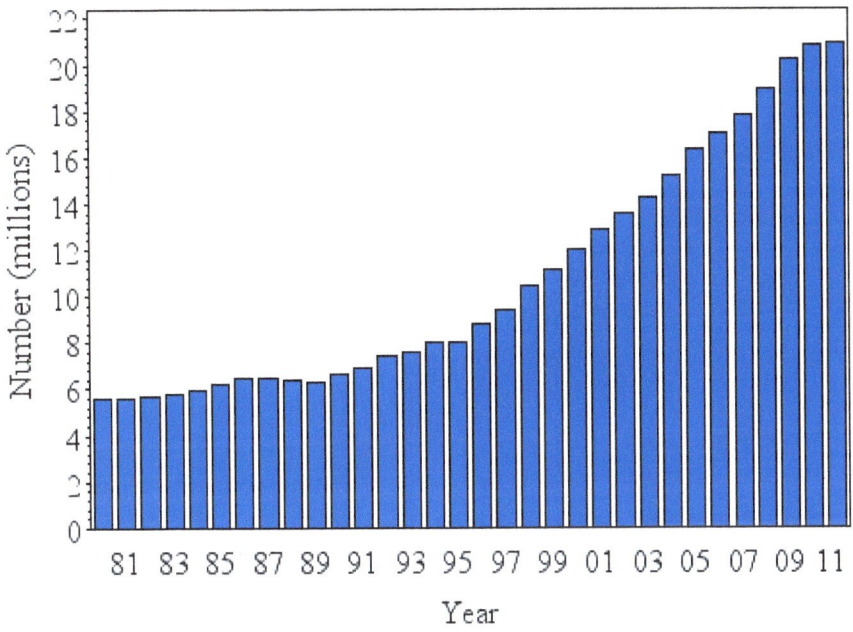

Figure 1-3- Total statin prescriptions by year

Statin prescriptions have exploded in the last 2 decades! The evidence behind this wild population study is very sketchy and, in many cases, negative. Prescriptions are up 10 x what they were 2 decades ago. ½ of our elderly population is in on the experiment. The bad news is that the newer guidelines will encourage your physicians to prescribe even more to even healthier people. Recent studies reveal that the risk for heart disease has been overestimated in men by between 37 and 154%! This means that many low risk patients will be/have been unnecessarily placed on these medications. As I will detail later, this is another failed experiment on the US population. The result is diabetes, memory loss and functional decline for many. The promise of longer life and fewer events is not delivered for the many. Sure, for those that have had heart attacks there is some evidence that there are fewer recurrent heart attacks, but what about for most people that are prescribed these medicines for prevention? These are the majority of people that were prescribed a statin medicine. Not someone just out of the ICU with a heart attack, but an otherwise relatively healthy person that feels fine except his doctor tells him his cholesterol number is too high? How do they do?

The answer is not very well. There have been 17 studies including 65,000 patients to study how effective these statin medicines are in primary prevention. Primary prevention means that you have not had a heart attack or stroke but are believed to be at risk for 1. To qualify, you must have at least one other known risk factor besides an elevated cholesterol. For example, these studies would include you if you have High blood pressure (hypertension), diabetes, are a smoker, or if you have a very strong family history for early heart attacks (age 55 or less) So how does primary prevention work in high risk patients? Answer, not well at all. Your chance of dying from a heart attack or stroke is unimproved. Isn't that one of the chief reasons to take the medicine? To prolong your life? Well a statin won't do that in primary prevention. In fact, it will lower your risk of a non-fatal heart attack a lowly 1.5 % and a stroke ½ %. Consider that many of these patients already have an extremely low risk to start with so that is a small percentage of a small percentage. And what about side effects? Oops, there is the dilemma, because for most they are worse than their risk. A full 10 % will get severe muscle issues, enough to discontinue therapy. I, myself was disabled by severe muscle cramps mandating the cessation of therapy and I have seen hundreds of others. On the surface muscle cramps may seem a minor side effect, but muscle function, strength and metabolism are important in the survival scheme.

Another side effect can be diabetes! Yes surprisingly 26% of those on a statin medicine develop diabetes when compared to a placebo. I will explain the probable mechanism behind the muscle damage and the development of diabetes later, but diabetes is a very serious condition! It is a leading cause of blindness, amputations, kidney failure, cardiovascular disease and death! Is it not ironic that a medicine that was designed to prevent cardiovascular events, in fact causes a condition which is possibly the most frequent cause of vascular events, diabetes!

There are other potential side effects of a statin medicine, memory loss is a common one. Your doctor may tell you that it is unrelated to the medicine, and that it is a natural process of aging, but I will detail why it can certainly be another ill effect of the medicine.

And now what about those very low risk patients? Those that don't' have any other risk factors yet? There are millions out there, that are otherwise healthy, that have been prescribed a statin medicine simply because their cholesterol number is too high, but they have no other risk factors. Their benefit shrinks to zero and their side effects predominate. I see these patients presenting to my office frequently. For example, a 30-year-old with only high cholesterol and they have parents and grandparents still alive with no family history of vascular disease. They have often a 20-40-year lead time that shows they are not at risk. Nonetheless their physician has insisted on a statin prescription to lower their infinitesimal risk. They will achieve none of the benefits and only side effects. With 30 million plus statin users out there, be assured that there are many non-risk patients out there who are dutifully taking the medicine.

So, are doctors and pharmaceutical companies the only ones in on the cholesterol scares? Even the government is in on the cholesterol scare. The pharmaceutical industry has the most lobbyist of any US industry. Billions of dollars are at stake. The government is involved in making guidelines. Pressure on our various leaders can influence the recommendations. It can influence the food our children get at school and dietary recommendations. Those in the know are alone against the food, medical, pharmaceutical and governments leaderships. This and ongoing new information is what motivated me to write my second book.

This gross misinformation reminds me of why I wrote my first book. It was this similar obsession by physicians, the food industry, and the government with cholesterol. It was the low-fat message... In the 1980's the medical profession came up with the idea that a high fat diet raises cholesterol, and of course, high cholesterol is a bad thing. This was one of the main points of my first book, "The globes best diet". The medical profession misleads the world based by its faulty and politically motivated interpretations of studies, and it sent the world (and especially the US) on an untested "low fat" diet. There was zero evidence to support this diet.

OOPS the experiment failed miserably! After 3 decades of this experiment, and with still with many patients religiously following this diet, we can see the results. Yes, the low-fat diet did lower cholesterol in some patients, but they did not see the reduced heart attacks and strokes that was predicated. In fact, they got more unhealthy! America has gotten progressively fatter in the last 3 decades! Now 2/3 of our population is overweight and 1/3 is obese Diabetes and pre-diabetes is exploding and there is no sign of reversal. I hate to inform you that the right fat is healthy, necessary, and essential. Our huge population experiment has failed, but nobody bothered to tell the patient, or for that matter the food industry!

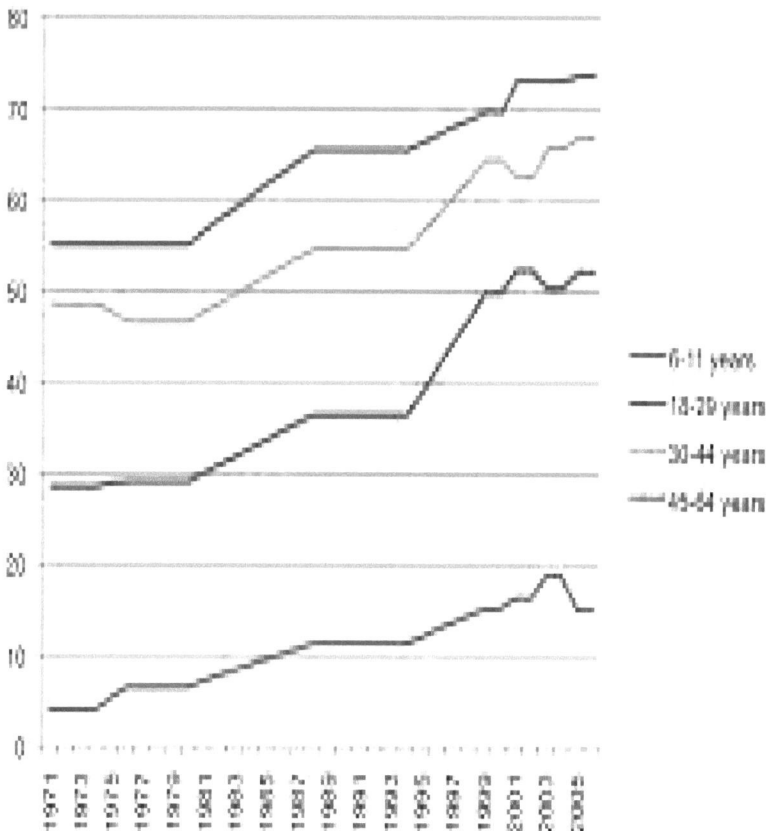

Figure 1-4 – Explosion of obesity on Low Fat diets

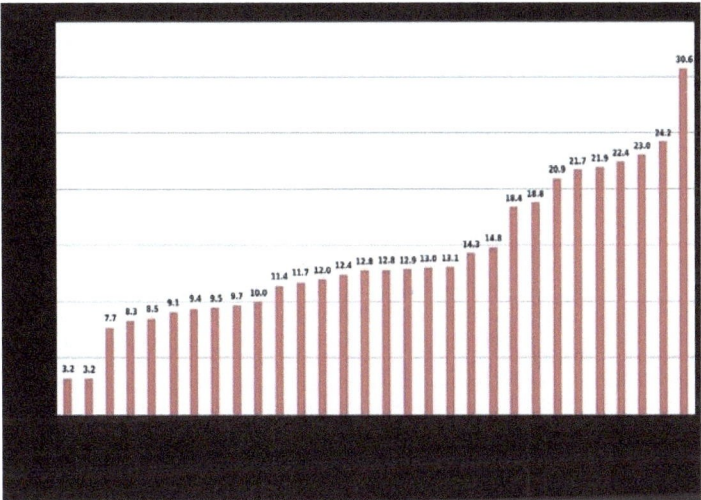

Figure 1-5 America is leading the way in obesity

How else can we lower cholesterol? How about if we change the fats. Let's see, if you cook with vegetable oil, it will lower your cholesterol "Mazola lowers cholesterol" That must be healthy. Soy lowers cholesterol, it must be healthy with its' Omega -6 fats. We'll talk more about this later, but this is another failed experiment. When I was in medical school, I learned that safflower oil was the best for lowering cholesterol, and of course that's good. Little did we know that we are poisoning our bodies with THESE fats, and not the fats that we were told avoid? Eat margarine, because it has less saturated fat and saturated fat raises cholesterol. It took medicine quite some time to discover that again, those who followed were poisoning their bodies with trans-fatty acids that were far worse than saturated fats. Our patients got unhealthier the harder they tried. This was also a main point in my first book "the globes best diet"

Low fat diet failed for another reason. 90% of the cholesterol in our body is produced in the liver and brain, not from dietary absorption. The body has internal mechanisms that control its production based on the demand for energy, hormones, nerve protection, food absorption etc. It will adjust its production based on the input or lack of input to attain its desired steady state, Diet has minimal effect on the end result.

The food industry jumped on this low-fat craze. Let's take the fat out of food. But wait, fat tastes good and if we take the fat out the food will taste bad. Hmm, what to do? I know take the fat out and add sugar! That tastes good! Here comes low fat milk, low fat pasta, low fat "protein bars" "low fat subway sandwiches" the list is endless. These sugar heavy foods turned out to be far worse than if we eat food in the natural state. But the food had another answer for sugar.

OOPs sugar is bad, hmmm. OK let's add this artificial sweetener. It tastes good and it contains no calories! That should be safe isn't it? Well, guess what, wrong again. These artificial sweeteners do not only not cause weight loss, but they caused more weight gain than if you used sugar instead! For each serving of an artificial sweetener (stevia excepted) there is 20% MORE weight gain per can! They increase your risk of diabetes and weight gain! How can this be? They have no calories. They are free drinks! The exact mechanism behind weight gain with something that has no calories is still ill-defined. My theory is that these non-digestible items slugs your metabolism, but that is only speculation. The problem with these diet drinks is that because they are "free" that people drink way more of them that they would if there were real sugar in them. I myself am a recovering diet cokeaholic. I would drink close to a 6 pack of the various flavors a day in my prime. What rational being would drink a 6 pack of regular coke, with its 900 calories in a day? Answer, an irrational fat one. But a 6 pack of zero calorie soda? Why not? What is the downside? The result is that many dieters gain even more weight than those than those that irrationally fat drinking the regular stuff. People trying to lose weight, and everybody needs to do that, are on this "low fat" diet- wrong again and are poisoning themselves also with artificial sweeteners. No wonder obesity is rampant in our society. Add in declining hormone levels (to be discussed later) and we have a full-blown obesity epidemic in place. Food has gone from nutritious and life giving to toxic!

So how have these diets fared for improving cholesterol? The answer is not good at all. Almost all diets have failed to lower cholesterol by any significant amount. As I will explain later, the idea that we have control over cholesterol levels is close to ridiculous. When there were minor changes in the cholesterol, the results were not what we expected. Although the total cholesterol did drop slightly with the low-fat diet, there was not the expected decline in heart disease. In, fact, people got more weight gain and diabetes and not less heart disease. The diet experiment failed, and America is the victims.

And what about the supposed goal? What are the glorified results of having "low cholesterol"? Not good. Very low cholesterol is associated with a higher risk for cancers and various infections.

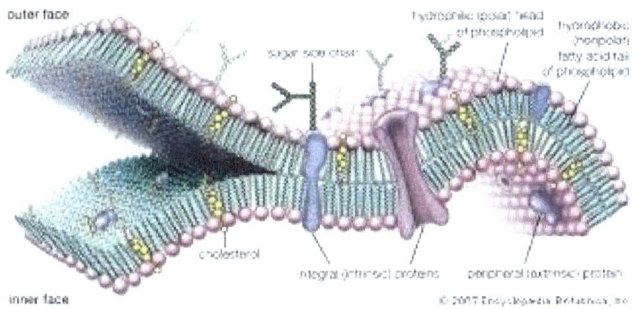

Figure 1-6

The circles on both sides of a cell wall represent cholesterol molecules. Every cell wall needs them to protect the cell from injury by infection, and toxins and cancer-causing agents. Cholesterol forms about ½ of all cell walls. The structure of cholesterol makes it perfect for forming cell walls. Everyone who has made a salad dressing knows that oil and water do not mix well. Cholesterol is the key balancing agent that allows the liquid blood to interact with the oilier protective cell walls. Cholesterol's chemical structure is uniquely designed for these purposes. It is known as an amphipathic molecule. That means is partially dissolvable in both water and oil.

Figure 1-7, Cholesterol structure

The left side of the molecule (the HO part) allows cholesterol to interact with water and blood. The hexagons give more solidity to the cell walls, and the CH_3 parts allow the cholesterol to mix with the oily inner components of the cell wall. The mixture allow cholesterol to be a barrier, yet to allow some movement through the walls

Low cholesterol is also associated with malnutrition. Most people don't' know that cholesterol is critical for food absorption. The liver converts cholesterol to bile acids, these are secreted in the bile during food digestion. Without these the body cannot absorb important body fats. Bile acids are also critical for absorption of fat soluble vitamins like vitamins A, D, E, and K. Low cholesterol could limit your supply of bile acids and impair food absorption, resulting in malnutrition.

Low cholesterol (levels of total cholesterol less than 160) has been linked to a higher risk for anxiety and depression. Cholesterol in cell walls is necessary to maintain the proteins that absorb the "happy hormone" serotonin, and people with low cholesterol have lower levels of serotonin. Some cholesterol medicines (especially lovastatin and simvastatin) are known to aggravate this issue, with associated worsening of mood issues... In fact, there is increased risk of violent, hostile and suicidal behaviors in those with low cholesterol, including low cholesterol that is chemically induced by certain statin medications. Low cholesterol is not what it is cracked up to be!

Low cholesterol may also be a risk factor for dementia, although studies are currently inconsistent in this category. Some studies suggest high cholesterol could be harmful, but many have shown just the opposite, that cholesterol is protective of development of dementia in elderly patients. Partial protection makes sense to me if you like at the figure below

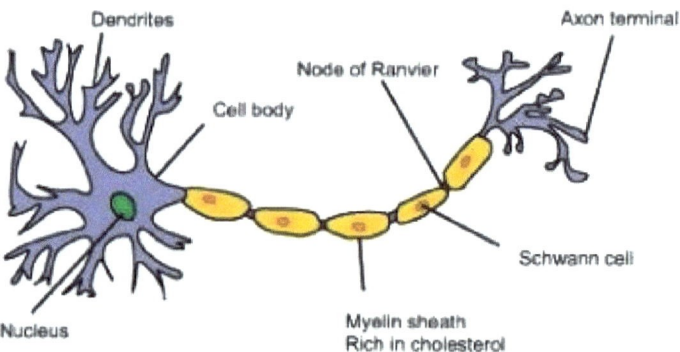

Figure 1-8 , Brain cell structure.

Brain cells have several parts, Critical to their function is the protection of axon, the long part that connects the nucleus to its target. The axon is surrounded by a cover, which is made largely of cholesterol. Without it the signals can be lost, and the nerve cell could be damaged. Progressive loss of nerve cells and nerve cell function could result in neurologic decline.

What else does cholesterol do? Cholesterol is the building block to produce many, life giving hormones.

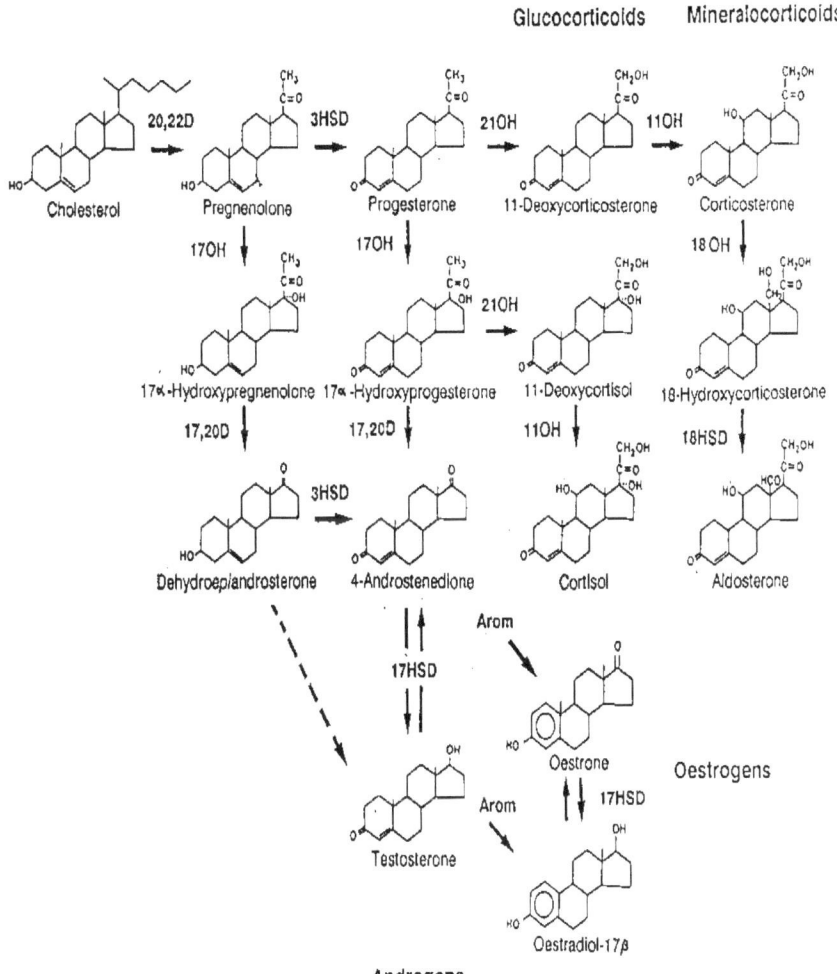

Figure 1-9, Cholesterol pathway to produce hormones

The above pathway is quite complicated, but it gives you an idea how necessary cholesterol is to produce CRTICAL hormones. Without cholesterol we could not have important hormones like cortisol, testosterone, estrogen, aldosterone, DHEA, pregnenolone, and progesterone. A full discussion of all these hormones is not possible in this text, but that life could not exist without them. These hormones serve many diverse functions. Deficiencies of them contributes to / causes many illnesses. In fact, complete lack of cortisol would cause death. Lower cholesterol would limit the basic ingredient needed to produce these critical hormones.

Also, amongst the hormones produced by cholesterol is pregnenolone. Most people have never heard of this key hormone, but it has been called the mother of all hormones.

It is the first step in conversion of cholesterol to other hormones. Not only is pregnenolone the mother of all hormones, it itself is a hormone, and more importantly a neurotransmitter. Its function is to improve mood and memory. Without cholesterol, and therefore without pregnenolone, you have CRS, can't remember Shinola. In other words, if you stop cholesterol production with a statin you stop production of pregnenolone and you can develop memory impairment like Alzheimer's disease. This is another mechanism that statin medicines could decrease memory function. If you take the medicine, you may forget to take the medicine!

Cholesterol metabolism is also critically involved in energy production.

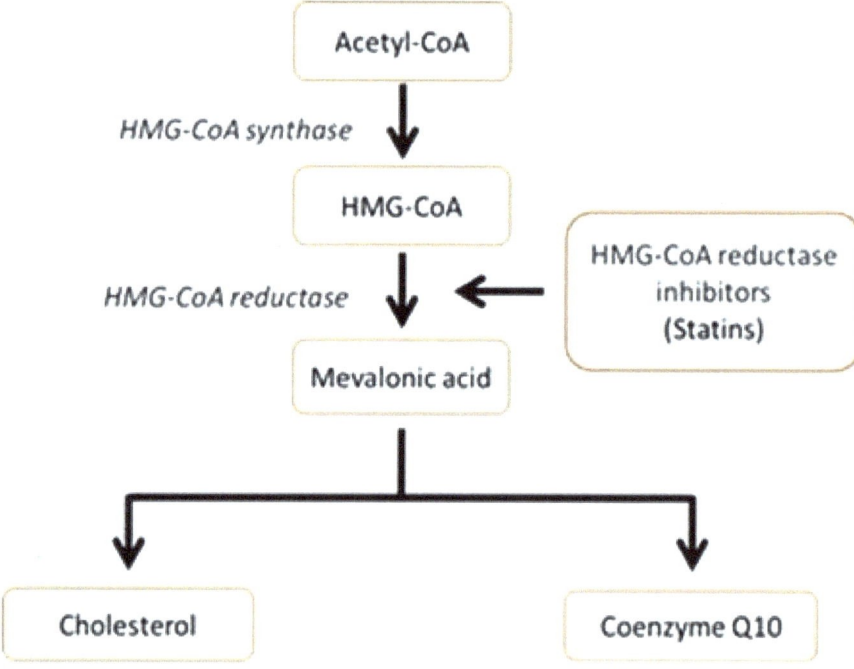

Figure- 1-10, Cholesterol formation. *Note that statins stop this production and with it the formation of coenzyme q 10.*

The building blocks that make cholesterol are critical ingredients to the energy production process. Co enzyme q 10, and its active metabolite ubiquinol are the limiting ingredients necessary for energy production. No cholesterol production results in no energy production! This could be the reason why patients put on statins are at higher risk of developing the lethal condition of diabetes. Without energy, the whole metabolic system starts to deteriorate. In fact, it has been shown that high potency statins like atorvastatin, decrease production of coenzyme q 10 in half! Coenzyme q 10 (and its resultant formation of energy) are critical for the function for the function of high demand energy requiring organs like muscle, the heart and brain. Statins are famous for causing muscle achiness and sometimes weakness. The lack of energy production may be instrumental in this. Isn't ironic that these medicines are mostly used to treat and prevent heart issues, yet they shutdown energy production in high energy organs like the heart!

Ubiquinol Declines With Age

Around age 40, we start losing Ubiquinol. This decline has been linked to accelerated aging and diminished energy levels.

Supplements can restore Ubiquinol to youthful levels.

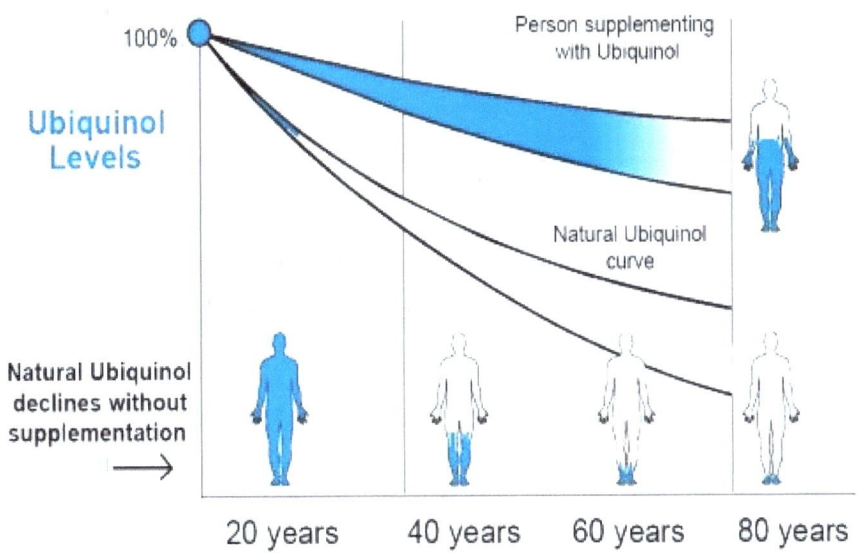

Figure 1-11, Ubiquinol levels with aging

Stopping the production of co q 10 only worsens the problems that already occurs with aging. Co q 10 levels drop drastically over time, with levels peaking when energy is best at age 20. We don't need a hastening of our energy decline, as is occurring with the addition of statins to our system. So, cholesterol is produced by the body for many important functions. It is important in the digestion process. It is critical in cell wall production. It is critical in the formation of many essential hormones. It is necessary to protect the brains neurons and preserve its function and it is critical for the energy production process. In short, we can't live without it!

So, what about its level, what should it be? The body has its own internal mechanism to determine this. The body has an internal signaling mechanism so if more cell walls are needed, if more hormones are needed, if cholesterol is needed for energy or for digestion, or for brain protection, then a signal is sent to the liver to produce more. The liver can assess how the supply based on ingestion and determine if more production is needed. We are jumping into this complex equation and we think we know better than the body that has been performing this delicate balance for 3 million years! How many cell walls do you need? Any physician that says he knows the answer to this question is a good liar. How much energy do you need? How many of each hormone do you need for optimal function? Medicine is only beginning to unravel these questions. The idea that we can control our cholesterol with diet or medicines is naïve! We don't' understand the body's internal mechanisms to jump into this. We can however keep your cholesterol happy! So, let's stop poisoning our bodies. I'll explain further how to live a healthy, happy productive life!

Chapter 2

AGING

We all know the symptoms of aging. They are so undoubtedly frozen in our brains and society. We expect a gradual decline in energy through each decade. Of course, you are getting older. That's expected. Then other things start to occur. Weight starts to appear around the midline. Sometimes there are obvious life style changes that contribute to it (ex. diminished activity, of course we have less energy, so activity is less) and at other times, this weight just appears gradually with no clear trigger. Most people are now aware that this weight gain in the middle is the start of something more sinister. It is a sign that there may be more serious underlying conditions ahead, but non-the-less, most people are powerless to stop the process.

Gradually, the symptoms get worse. The mood isn't what it used to be. The bright cheerful moods are intermittently spaced now with a shortened fuse. Moods can be irritable and grumpy at times, if not even depressed. Anxiety over minor issues becomes more prevalent. This can progress to outright panic attacks. Some people are spared this more than others, but already by the 30's many people are already taking Prozac or Xanax for mood disturbances. Within a few decades these initial mood changes can progress to grumpy old men and raging menopausal women. All normal right?

The age train doesn't stop there however, no unfortunately it gets much worse. Now the sexual identity begins to fade. The sexuality that drove us in our teens and early 20's starts to slip. For men the libido starts to diminish, and the erections gradually become more difficult and less fulfilling. For women their drive and responsiveness also decline, and along with it, the marriages and relationships that are founded on it. Temporarily a partner can be blamed for the decline and solutions are sought outside of the relationship. This can result in another complication of aging, Divorce.

The "age train" still relentlessly continues. Sleep, which in the past was always refreshing becomes more strained. Getting to sleep and staying asleep can become a struggle. Even if a full night of sleep is garnered, it may not have comprised the restful rejuvenating sleep that was present in earlier years. Instead, you may now awake tired and resort to coffee, sugar foods, and energy drinks to provide the needed energy boosts. Little do you know that longer term this will only worsen the problem. Sleep aids appear, first the over the counter ones which provide more time in bed, but not restful sleep. Then attempted self –medication with alcohol for sleep might appear. Eventually a trip to the doctor for a prescription fix to sleep issues. Ambien,

Lunesta, or any of the other pharmaceutical wonders may provide some temporary relief, but at an unknown cost. Sleep may be longer, but not restful and healing. In fact, many patients feel drugged or hungover the next morning, and as I will elucidate later, they are further depriving themselves of the body's natural sleep and repair mechanisms (melatonin) and longer term only aggravating the "aging" process.

It may take 20 years or longer for the final phases to develop. The disease train has arrived. That dangerous belly fat has now accumulated to the point that it is affecting your health in a noticeable manner. The blood sugar starts to elevate, at first gradually and imperceptibly, but it marches relentlessly. At this point you are unaware that inflammation has taken a deep seat in your system. The belly fat will be accompanied by a rise in Triglycerides. Triglycerides are the other body fat that is transported in the blood besides cholesterol. It signals a sugar overload in the system as does the belly fat and elevating blood sugar. As a part of this process, blood pressure can also elevate. The body becomes so accustomed to sugar challenges that is loses its sensitivity to them and it must release more and more insulin to achieve the same process. This insulin resistance, abdominal fat, elevated triglycerides and blood pressure elevations together are termed the metabolic syndrome. The metabolic syndrome is a rampant pre-diabetic condition in our society, but for most, that belly fat is just aging.

Once we have gotten to this phase of health, the downward decline proceeds more rapidly. The inflammation in the system multiplies. This inflammation becomes symptomatic. The joints start to ache and get stiff. Arthritis is developing now. This is part of the normal aging process, right? This should be expected? For some, the combination of extra belly weight and joint inflammation starts a vicious cycle. The extra weight puts more pressure on the joints which are already inflamed. This gravitational stress further inflames the joints so that the solution for many is to further limit activity. This promotes more weight gain, which further aggravates inflammation and gravitational pressure. We are headed to a knee replacement at 50 now.

The age train continues. As the inflammation builds up, the bodies structures get further damaged. Key of these is the mitochondria. The body's cells have certain parts, and one of the most important is the mitochondria. The mitochondria are the body's energy factories. 95% of the body's energy are produced in the mitochondria! There function is vital for your survival. They provide the energy for your heart to contract and send blood to other parts of the body. They provide the energy necessary for the thought process, and they provide the energy for your body to repair. The also provide the energy needed to fight off inflammation. They like other body parts, can also get inflamed and be injured by that process. The result is a worsened metabolism of energy. This now is the faster road to decline. As energy production diminishes. So, does the efficiency of all body organs. For the mitochondria, this may be reflected in even poorer metabolism of sugar, this pre-diabetic condition is now progressing to full blown diabetes, with all its toxic ramifications. As their function in cells decline, so does the function of the organs they serve. Now the aging and inflammatory process has progresses to full blown diseases.

This inflammatory process can also attack proteins. Proteins are part of the body's metabolic process that is necessary for the body to metabolize food, generate energy, detoxify and repair itself. These proteins can be irreversible injured by the inflammatory process with a gradual decline in their function. The daily functions are thus slowing down and becoming more inefficient or even non-functional as these proteins are progressively injured.

Both the inside and outsides   are damaged by the age train externally the skin becomes damaged, but the inflammation caused by light exposure and the inflammation that is occurring from within. Now skin discolorations, wrinkles and other physical signs of aging become apparent. The age is now apparent in the mirror, certainly this is normal?

The age process continues and with it, now more diseased develops. In the arteries an inflammatory process begins. At first this inflammation is like tiny dents on a new car. Visibly minor or imperceptible, but perhaps noticeable to that new car owner. As more and more inflammatory insults attack the arteries, the flow of blood gets disrupted by the wall imperfections. This flow disturbance can lead to further damage and inflammations that can result in a progressive process. This" normal again process" is termed atherosclerosis, and it can eventually result in complete loss of circulation to the affected part. Heart attacks strokes, leg amputations and kidney failure are some of the "expected" parts of aging.

The age train continues now to the depths of illness. The inflammation now attacks the control panel DNA. DNA controls what the cell produces, it controls which proteins are produced for health and metabolism. It also controls whether a cell will divide itself. When DNA is damaged, the control mechanism can become broken, the signal to multiply can go array, and then the possibility of cancer develops. Normally the body can further control this with the immune system that will ward off unwanted cells or organisms. Unfortunately, the immune system has also been damaged by the inflammation and it is unable to control the new growth. It is also less able to fight off infections like pneumonia, influenza and others.

The inflammatory process continues in the brains and the memory becomes less sharp, and soon recent events become poorly recorded, as it progresses nerves are permanently injuring, and the process of permanent memory loss or so-called Alzheimer's dementia are in progress. Eventually a summation of these injuries leads to the worst sign of aging Death of the organism. At the time of this writing, eventual death is still a fact of life, but the age progressions above can be slowed or even reversed with the right methods. I will show you how you can get off the age trains and move yourself to a healthier, happier, disease Free State in my ensuring chapter.

Chapter 3

OXIDATION/INFLAMMATION

Part 1 Oxidation Oxygen is essential for life. It is its reactivity that creates energy itself. It is the transfer of electrons from oxygen to coenzyme Q 10 to form the energy rich ubiquinol which is at the center of energy production. This metabolic process is performed in the bodies metabolic and energy factories, the mitochondria. It must have oxygen to complete the process. Oxygen is the second most electron negative element. In other words, it is freer to give away free electrons than almost any other element. It is its generosity with electrons that allows energy production. Without it, humans and can only survive a matter of minutes before we are unable to meet our huge energy requirements. In other words, the dying process begins as soon as oxygen energy generation is shut off. Without oxygen we would not exist nor survive. When the process works properly, we can utilize this source of energy to supply all our bodies needs for the activities of life. Our motions, thinking, circulation, and defense against the environment all require energy. A limitation of its supply will cause a progressive decline of bodily functions, with the eventual result of death! Without efficient Oxygen supply and utilization, we are sunk sooner or later. So that's the good news on Oxygen, without it, we die, we need it for everything, now for the bad news, 98% of the time, oxygen reacts according to plan and produces energy without a glitch. Go life! But then, there is the other 2%. In this case the electrons just don't go where they are supposed to. Electrons are a without loyalty. They have no mind and don't really care where they go, they just want someone to accept them as they are not very good in the single state. They want to marry. Their preferable marriage partner is ubiquinol, but in any given second they will attach to whoever is conveniently located. Jilted from marriage, the electron becomes an indiscriminating whore! Here is where the trouble starts. The body has well defined structures that function perfectly in their original state, but they don't function nearly as well when that structure is altered, even by as much as an electron. This jilted electron will grab onto whatever structure is closest. This creates an instability in this "oxidized" molecule. Usually this molecule is not designed to handle the excess electron, so this new molecule is itself unstable. Not only is it unstable, but the electron can affect the structure of the new "oxidized molecule" in a way that its function is diminished or non-functional. This new molecule is then unstable, and the result can be a chain reaction. One unstable molecule then attaches and attacks another molecule and so on. It is thought that this progressive damage from oxygen byproducts (so called reactive oxygen species or ROS for short) that is at the center of aging, disease and death!

This process can occur anywhere in the body. There is no body part that is immune to the aging process and oxidative damage. It occurs most frequently where oxygen is at work, in the mitochondria. This is where 95% of the body's energy is produced. As oxygen injures these organelles, there can be a progressive loss of energy production. Since all body functions require energy, this progressive loss of energy production produces widespread consequences in the body's ability to function and fight off disease. This oxidative process then initiates a further inflammatory process that further injures the surrounding tissues. The mitochondrial theory is that all illnesses start with decline in the energy production system and inflammatory damage that predominately occurs within the body's energy factories the mitochondria. In other words, Oxygen gives us the energy of life, but consequently it produces the byproducts that cause death!

This same process also occurs wherever oxygen is, and in the human body, that is everywhere by necessity. One way that this damage becomes more obvious is the development of cardiovascular disease. This is how the term "bad cholesterol" came about. LDL- or so called "bad cholesterol" is produced in the liver in response to the bodies needs for cholesterol. It is released in beautifully packaged floating vehicles. The cholesterol molecule is specifically designed for this transport. Its structures are amphipathic. In laymen terms, it is a molecule that equally loves fat and water. That makes it an ideal molecule to transport things through the blood yet enable to find a place to rest comfortably in fat tissues or usually on the margins between both! It is a truly miraculous structure! LDL-cholesterol is such a floating package. The system works quite beautifully until along comes an unmarried electron that has escaped. This unstable electron can then attach to LDL cholesterol, which itself then becomes unstable. This is cholesterol gone bad. This instability can result in LDL-cholesterol attaching itself to other structures, like the blood vessel wall. This process can become irreversible if the electron is not neutralized quickly. This action can occur over and over in someone's lifetime. After endless years of oxidative damage, the wall can get compressed and more unstable. Eventually the instability and circulatory compromise results in loss of oxygen to other tissues, and further damage occurs. The result is cardiovascular disease with its complications, heart attacks, strokes and death. The point is however. CHOLESTEROL IS FOUND AT THE SCENE OF THE CRIME, BUT NOT THE PERPETRATOR OF THE CRIME! The criminal is the free electrons that damage the structures to begin with, in other words, the oxidative process.

Oxygen and the instability it creates, goes on throughout the body. Another key is in our own DNA. DNA gives our body the code it need to function properly. It is critical that this code remain intact. Minor changes in this code can result in everything from poor body function to cancer and death. When oxygen, and its undesired metabolites touch DNA, the free electrons can disrupt the structure of DNA. DNA is our master control panel. Disruption here can have widespread consequences. Of concern is that alteration of the control mechanism can result in cancer. The body's directions have been lost to randomness. Other body organ function will also suffer for lack of the normal control panel instructions and this can result in progressive loss of function and further "aging'

Aging is really the progressive decline of bodily function that we see when oxidative damage permanently injures the healthy functioning body. Cholesterol, like other bodies structures like DNA and mitochondria are injured in the process but are not the causes of the injury. They just happened to be in the wrong place at the wrong time.

Other factors can promote inflammation in your body besides a high sugar, high omega 6 diet. Smoking is a major contributor to inflammation and it is a major reason for its widespread damage. Obesity, partially mediated by abdominal fat is a contributor. Sleep deprivation cause inflammation, Stress and over-exercise are also aggravating factors

Now that we have identified 1 of the real enemies. In subsequent chapters I will discuss how to fight and win and against this opponent.

Chapter 4

GLYCATION-

Sugar is everywhere these days. There is the natural sugar present in foods. If you listen to the USDA, 40% of your diet should be in sugary grains.

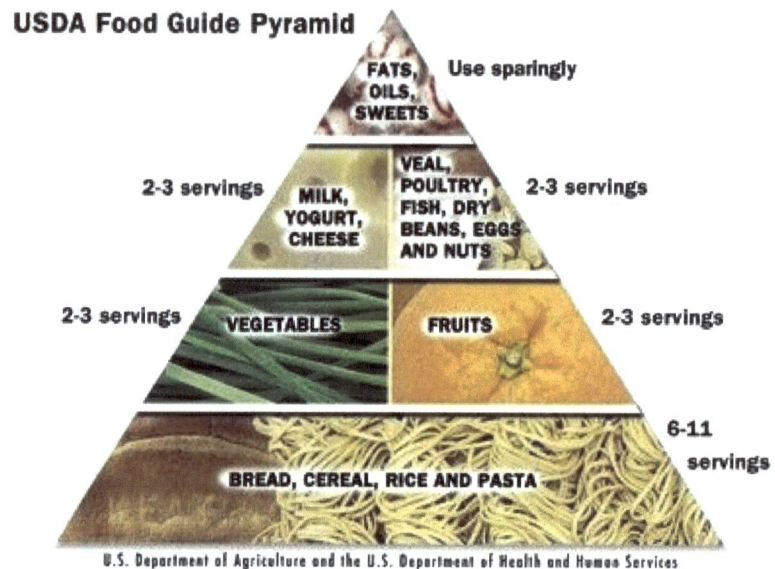

USDA Food Guide Pyramid

FATS, OILS, SWEETS — Use sparingly

2-3 servings — MILK, YOGURT, CHEESE

VEAL, POULTRY, FISH, DRY BEANS, EGGS AND NUTS — 2-3 servings

2-3 servings — VEGETABLES

FRUITS — 2-3 servings

BREAD, CEREAL, RICE AND PASTA — 6-11 servings

U.S. Department of Agriculture and the U.S. Department of Health and Human Services

Figure 3-1, USDA food pyramid which emphasizes carb rich foods

That should be bad enough, but most people don't follow the food pyramid. If you notice processed foods like sodas, candies, so called "protein bars", are additional sources of these toxic molecules. What is the body requirement for sugar? According to the USDA 40% of your nutrition should come from sugar, but the body requirement for external sugar is ZERO! You can make all the sugar you need internally.

Besides oxidation, and it's resultant inflammation. The sugar molecule itself is the other enemy to the stability (homeostasis or stable condition) of the body. That process of sugar damage to the system is glycation. Glycation is being attacked and damaged by a sugar molecule. Violent sugar molecules? Who knew? It turns out that there are several types of sugar Glycation.

Sugar is the enemy, not cholesterol. Sugar has various forms. Many people say, I don't eat any sugar. By that they mean table sugar. How wrong they are! Sugar is the general term for a short carbohydrate molecule. They

can exist as their basic units called monosaccharides. There are 3 possibilities, glucose (also known as dextrose) fructose, and galactose. Interestingly, they all have the same chemical formula, but they arranged slightly different
They can combine with each other and form 2 sugar molecules, called disaccharides. Sucrose or table sugar is combination of glucose and fructose. Maltose is 2 glucose molecules, Lactose or milk sugar is combination of galactose and sucrose.

Sugar molecules can also combine to form long chains, or so called complex carbohydrates.

Figure 3-2, The chemical structure of fructose

Sugars are unstable molecules, they contain 6 oxygen molecules. Each O above represents an oxygen molecule. Oxygen helps create energy because it can donate its electrons in the energy production process. It is chemically unstable and that is both the good and the bad news. The good news is that this instability allows energy production, the bad news is this instability can also be toxic. These electrons can grab onto any structure that it encounters. There is another word for sugar molecules binding to other chemical structure that word is AGING!

The sugar molecules can enter the blood and here is where some of the toxicity begins. A common example of this toxicity is hemoglobin A 1 c. basically this is a hemoglobin molecule, the one that carries oxygen that is bound to hemoglobin. When sugar in the blood encounters the hemoglobin, the sugar can permanently latch on to the hemoglobin. That hemoglobin becomes non-functional in the carrying of oxygen. The percentage of hemoglobin that is non –functional and permanently attached to glucose in the blood can be measured and is called hemoglobin A1c. It is used in medicine to monitor diabetes, but non- diabetics are also susceptible to this form of damage. How much do you want to damage your system with glucose? How much oxygen do you want to deprive your system of? The correct answer is the less the better!

Sugar toxicity can go way beyond damaging to hemoglobin and thereby oxygen consumption and energy production. Sugar molecules of all kinds still contain those 6 oxygen molecules that are chemically unstable in the human body. They are just full of those single electrons that want to grab onto anything. Enter another complication of aging AGE, or advance glycation end products.

When a sugar molecule binds to other structures in the body, it can form irreversible bonds with the sugar molecule attached to what was previously a normally functioning molecule. It can bind to any protein or enzyme, now rendering that enzyme non-functional. Any of the sugar molecules can do this, sucrose, fructose, galactose, ectara. At first this binding can be reversible. The sugar can bind to the protein and then be released from it. In general, the presence of vitamin B6(pyridoxine) is required to allow reversibility of this process. If the process does not reverse, IT CAN PROGRESS! The protein can get further linked to the sugar molecule, permanently damage it, and then initiate a further inflammatory response. This combination of sugar molecules bound to, and irreversibly damaging body tissues like proteins is called advanced glycation endpoints (AGE) Basically, there are piles of sugar and their attacked body components that just start to build up in your system! Once the process starts, a secondary inflammatory reaction develops, further aggravating the issue. The accumulation of these products can then disable the cells function and start the cell death process. We are then dying/aging, protein by protein, and cell by cell, in a progressive heap of sugar garbage! It is the accumulation of these byproducts that is that be underlie degenerative disease processes like diabetes, atherosclerosis, Alzheimer's disease and others. Diabetes itself is a disease of accelerated aging.

Besides eating the sugar that causes this process, we can cook in our AGE. Foods like meats and butter have them already. We can also produce these sugar protein junk piles in the cooking process. Dry cooking produces the most damage. The cooking methods of frying, roasting, grilling or baking, produces these AGE, which we then ingest and absorb into our system.

Boiling, steaming, microwaving, and stewing are cooking methods that produce fewer AGE's. Try to cook at lower heat, for shorter time periods, and add lemon or vinegar to minimize the AGE production and absorption into your system

You can also smoke you AGE's. The burning of tobacco introduces the burnt sugar molecules into your system. Just another reason not to smoke,

Sugar can bind to DNA, and now that DNA can no longer divide normally. In fact, it's structure can change so much, that if it does divide, it may divide abnormally and create a cancer cell! Therefore, diabetics can get much higher risk of many cancers. There is sugar toxicity to DNA that disrupts the process. Diabetics have up to double the risk of some forms of cancer, and it is likely this sugar toxicity to DNA is at the root.

Sugar molecules can also bind to fats (lipids) like cholesterol. When a sugar irreversibly binds to a fat, it is called and ALE (advanced lipid end) These can accumulate in the blood vessels and combined with the resultant inflammatory process. They can initiate the hardening of the artery process that has been blamed on its victim. Cholesterol. Cholesterol is found at the scene of the crime, but not the perpetrator of the crime, the criminal in this case, is the sugar molecule. The sugar molecule (because of its instability) combines with the LDL-cholesterol (so called bad cholesterol) and then damages it. The result is a progressive accumulation of fatty junk particle.

There has been much speculation as to which type of sugar molecule is the worst. Remember, they all have the same chemical structure. They can all initiate the processes above, including the development of AGE and ALE and aging. They can have different effects on metabolism however, in their normal, non- attacking state.

Most would think that fructose, the sugar derived predominately from fruit, would be preferable to dextrose (found in cookies pies, etc.) and galactose (found mostly in milk products) At first glance, most people would choose the fruit sugar (fructose) to be less likely to cause damage than the dextrose and galactose. Here, the source matters. If the fructose is derived from its natural source, (i.e. a whole fruit or vegetable) there are some counter balancing nutrients, like anti-oxidants, vitamins and fiber that add nutritional value and protection to the sugar. Yes, choose the whole fruit over a glass of milk, or a cupcake, Easy. But what about fructose by itself (as in soft drinks or many processed foods) and in high quantities? Not so good. Besides the toxicity of the sugar molecule itself, fructose is metabolized differently than the other sugars. This altered digestion/ metabolism can have profound effects on health.

Anyone who still insists that "sugar is sugar" is way behind the times... There are in fact major differences in how your body processes different sugars, and it's important to understand that when you consume fructose, your body packs on pounds at a much higher rate than it does when you consume glucose. The following summary details the main metabolic differences between fructose and glucose to help you understand how fructose can wreak such havoc with your health, and why it's considerably worse for you than glucose:

- After eating fructose, nearly all the metabolic burden rests on your liver. But with glucose, your liver must break down only 20 percent.
- Every cell in your body, including your brain, utilizes glucose. Therefore, much of it is "burned up" immediately after you consume it. By contrast, fructose is primarily converted into free fatty acids (FFAs), VLDL (the damaging form of cholesterol), and triglycerides, which get stored as fat.
- The fatty acids created during fructose metabolism accumulate as fat droplets in your liver and skeletal muscle tissues, causing insulin resistance and non-alcoholic fatty liver disease (NAFLD). Insulin resistance progresses to metabolic syndrome and type II diabetes.
- When you eat 120 calories of glucose, less than one calorie is stored as fat. 120 calories of fructose results in 40 calories being stored as fat. Fructose is essentially largely converted into fat!
- The metabolism of fructose by your liver creates a long list of waste products and toxins, including a large amount of uric acid, which triggers your "fat switch," causing you to gain more weight.
- Glucose does not do this, as it suppresses the hunger hormone ghrelin and stimulates leptin, which suppresses your appetite. Fructose has no effect on ghrelin and interferes with your brain's communication with leptin, resulting in overeating

In summary, all sugar is toxic. Processed foods that concentrate fructose are the most dangerous as they promote more weight gain, insulin resistance, and stress on your metabolism.

Now that we have identified the real enemies, let's go on to what you can do to protect yourself from the enemies of oxidation and glycation. The options include proper diet, nutritional supplement and hormone optimization as your path the win against the age train and love your cholesterol!

Chapter 5

THE PALEO DIET

The Paleo diet is the one that man survived on before the advent of advanced agricultural techniques, the advent of food processing and the supplementation with animal dairy products. It goes like this

Eat NONE of the following

Grain products – All grains including whole grain products, cereals, breads, pasta, oatmeal, rice, etc.

Dairy products

Legumes- All beans, lentils, soy, kidney, peanuts, exceptions green beans and snow peas

Starches –Potatoes and Corn

Processed foods

Sugar, alcohol, salt

Vegetable oils

Eat and Enjoy the following-

Grass feed meats – Beef, Pork, lamb, organ meats

Turkey chicken, eggs

Wild caught seafood

Vegetable herbs and spices (not potatoes, sweet potatoes, or corn)

Fruit (especially berries and citrus)

Nuts and seed (except peanuts and cashews)

INCREASE intake of

Root vegetables – carrots, turnips. Beets, rutabagas

Organ meats -Liver, kidney, heart

Cave man had it right! God provided us with all the natural and nutritious food, we just must eat it. Our survival attests to its effectiveness. He had none of the processed foods. Agriculture was not developed yet, so large amounts of grain products as encouraged by our government was not possible. As far as dairy goes, it appears that dairy products entered our society only in the last 5000 years or so with breeding of goats, camels, and later cows. We are the only animal that drinks another animals milk. We forget that milk is designed to provide RAPID GROWTH to the babies that ingest it. Is that the goal of our readers? To rapidly expand body size? I think not. Much attention has been put to the fat content of milk, little to its sugar content. Milk is a high fat high sugar food and therefore has the toxicity of sugar in it. 46% of the calories from low fat milk are sugar derived. Even whole milk is 1/3 sugar! What makes matters worse is the type of sugar. Milks main sugar is lactose, which is difficult for many to digest. Gas, belly pain, and bloating are the unexpected and often hidden complications of milk ingestion. And what about calcium? Don't you need milk for all that calcium and vitamin D? Milk does a body good right? Doesn't it build strong bones? Recent studies have suggested the opposite. There was HIGHER bone fracture risk in milk drinkers! Even worse, higher milk consumption lead to a higher risk of DYING! Milk does not do a body good, it promotes fracture and death, and in my book, those aren't good outcomes. I will circle back to the Vitamin D requirements later in this book but suffice it to say now that the 100 units of vitamin D in milk are miniscule compared to our requirements and not worth the sugar, bone and life damage to warrant drinking milk for this purpose.

Beans are more controversial in the paleo diet. Many view beans as healthy foods, including soy which was touted as health food in recent decades. Large amounts of bean products are dependent on agriculture, which is still only a recent addition to human survival. They were not a large part of the diet and they have some surprisingly negative health consequences. One of the downside to beans is their sugar content. They are moderately high is sugar, which we know now is toxic. The types of fats in soybeans is also undesirable. They are very high in Omega6 fatty acids. The body can process 2 main types of fats, omega 3 (which are found in fish) and omega-6, found in beans. The omega-6 does provide energy, but it feeds a metabolic chain that tends to promote inflammation, whereas omega 3 sources tend to do the opposite, to reduce inflammation. About ½ of the fat in soybeans is the pro-inflammatory omega 6 variety. Over time this can lead to a progression of inflammation and the achy old body we are trying to avoid.

Another issue with beans (and grains) is Phytic Acid. Seeds, bran (including oat bran) and soybeans are the highest in phytic acid. They are highly indigestible unless fermented. Phytic acid is present in these foods and it is a nutrient deplete. By itself it binds phosphorous along with other essential minerals like calcium, magnesium, iron and zinc and make them unavailable for absorption. The body critically needs these elements for metabolism and body function. Besides impairing mineral absorption, they also bind to digestive enzymes that digest sugar and protein. This can decrease their nutritional value and the value of other foods eaten. The result of high intake is osteoporosis in adults and short stature and rickets in children.

There is another side to this coin. Paleo and ketogenic diets restrict beans. What do the studies show? Beans were restricted partially because of high sugar content. The proponents of beans cite their very low glycemic index. (this measure shown tightly the sugar is bound to fiber, lower reading suggests they are bound and therefore the sugar will be more slowly released and not cause the insulin surge and weight gain expected) They do, in fact, have low glycemic index. How do they perform in studies?

Surprisingly well! In 1 study, they lowered average blood sugar reading and weight, which are my main concerns for beans. In another study, centenarians reported bean intake as one of their main nutrients! In a Japanese study, beans were shown to decrease cardiovascular disease and prolong life. So, we have the theory of harm to weight and blood sugar, not substantiated in limited studies. We have studies supporting their promotion of longevity. Which way do you vote? To bean or not to bean?

In my opinion it is an individual decision. Certainly, if you do eat beans, you would want to minimize any harm by proper handling. This includes soaking, then draining, then cooking (not slowly) then draining. This is too much for many. Canned beans have Bisphosphenal A, which is toxic.

Even with proper preparation, those with GI disorders or auto-immune disorders should avoid them. As they are high in sugar content, there is caution for diabetics or those concerned about weight (who isn't?) On the positive side, there has been a study that showed these sugar and weight fears may be overdone. Longevity studies appear to be in beans favor.

Bottom line, I would not go out of my way to add these into your diet, and they may be acceptable for some patients in moderation, if not even health promoting with proper preparation. Eat cautiously.

The main reason that you might consider this nutrient is if you have a very high protein intake. High protein intake does have a correlation to cancer and cardiovascular disease. Certainly, protein is not as toxic as sugar, but there are some risks. Overall the paleo will help greatly for weight control and diabetes prevention because of the lower sugar content, but if your paleo focus is more on meats than on vegetables, nuts, and fruits, beans might be a way to minimize protein overload. There have been studies to show healthy populations can survive on much lower protein intake than an average American. Cautious substitution, may minimize the risks in some.

As far as grains go, many are surprised that their beloved grain products, even the whole grain products are on the do not eat list. Whole grain bread, for example is 80% sugar! Oatmeal is 74% sugar! Brown rice is 85% sugar! We already know that sugar is a toxic molecule. Critics will say that the sugar is bound to essential fiber which slows the sugar absorption and itself provided some health benefits. True, the proper kind of fiber can improve the digestive process. Remember however that grains contain phytates, which then also has an anti-digestive component. Fiber slows absorption of sugar, so you get less of a sugar rush, and therefore less insulin surge and less weight gain than with a processed sugar. Forced to eat a whole grain product or a processed grain, I will choose the whole grain product. The bottom line however, is that sugar, in whatever vehicle, is still sugar and has the potential for toxicity to your system and its resultant acceleration of aging. It none-the-less provides non-essential sugar calories. They are otherwise lacking in most nutrients like vitamins and critical anti-oxidants which are required to handle the toxic sugar molecule.

What about fats? Many high fat foods were not readily available in the paleo period. Because they were not broadly available in the paleo period, does that prove that they are unhealthy? I think not. Omega 3's were not available to land locked paleo man, does that prove they are unhealthy? No, they are quite the opposite. Who is to say that the paleo diet was an optimal diet for humans. We survived with is, but does that make it optimal for health?

Take the case of some of these fats, Coconut oil, olive oil, abundant avocados or avocado oil, cheeses, Greek yogurt, MCT oil, cream, butter and more. These are all have very low or absent sugar contents (the main enemy) They are also not overladen with protein which has its risk. Some of them have the less desirable forms of sugar that could promote GI distress but are otherwise clean from a nutrient standpoint.

Studies have shown fats to be the least harmful of the 3 macros, sugar, protein, and fats. It turns out high fat content lowers the risk of cardiovascular disease and death! Why? Fat is the cleanest burning energy source. It doesn't have toxic sugar, and much fewer if any oxygen molecules. It can produce energy without many of the toxic inflammatory by-products that sugar produces. These are excluded from the typical paleo diet, despite their health attributes.

In summary, I don't think that a foods absence is de-novo proof of its harm, let's consider the data. I would postulate that a healthier diet would be the love your cholesterol diet as this.

Eat NONE of the following

Grain products – All grains including whole grain products, cereals, breads, pasta, oatmeal, rice, etc.

 Reduced fat dairy products

Starches –Potatoes and Corn

Processed foods

Sugar, alcohol, salt

Vegetable oils

Eat and Enjoy the following-

Grass feed meats – Beef, Pork, lamb, organ meats

Turkey chicken, eggs

Wild caught seafood

Vegetable herbs and spices (not potatoes, sweet potatoes, or corn)

Fruit (especially berries and citrus)

Nuts and seed (except peanuts and cashews)

Fats- Coconut oil, olive oil, MCT oil, cheese, cream, butter, avocado oil, Greek yogurt consider adding these into your diet

INCREASE intake of

Root vegetables – carrots, turnips. Beets, rutabagas Organ meats -Liver, kidney, heart

*Legumes- All beans, lentils, soy, kidney, peanuts, exceptions green beans and snow peas- in moderation (must be properly prepared, not for those with GI issues or auto-immune disorders, caution in diabetes or weight issues)

Chapter 6

HORMONES

Now that you have learned how to stop poisoning your body with sugar and inflammation to slow the age decline, how do we start to reverse the process? The answer is in hormones. The body has innumerable hormones. Many of these are critical if not essential for life. For example, type I Diabetes is complete absence of the hormone insulin. This condition was universally lethal before the isolation of insulin for administration. Thyroid deficiency (hypothyroid) is lethal if severe and untreated. Testosterone deficiency causes a severe decline in health resulting in fatal conditions. Estradiol (the active form of the predominately female hormone estrogen) deficiency (called menopause in women) leads to severe health decline eventually resulting in death. Deficiency of only 1 of the key hormones can be sufficient to cause severe decline in quality of life and health eventually resulting in death.

Hormones are different in their action site is different than where most medications have their activity. Medications and supplements act in the cytoplasm or basically the body of the cell. A hormone is structure that acts on the DNA, so it can modify the bodies function and composition. Enzymes and medications cannot interact with DNA to change the body. Hormones are therefore more powerful! They are the secret control panel that has the ability to change you, not just band-aid you like medications.

All hormones have their specific functions Not all of them have antiaging properties. There are a few that do have that effect, or research suggests that. Amongst them are testosterone, estradiol, growth hormone, and growth hormone similar IGF-1. I will focus on the anti-aging properties of testosterone and estradiol, as discussion of some of the other hormones is beyond the scope of this book.

The word hormone comes from the Greek work Hormon, which means to set in motion, excite, or stimulate. Some people may be surprised that hormones have anti-aging properties, but let's start with energy. People associate the gradual decline of energy with age. The truth is that hormonal decline can also cause identical symptoms. The fatigue commonly associated with deficiencies of hormones like testosterone and estradiol can be perfectly reversed with optimal hormone replacement! Isn't it great that you don't have to live with an ancient person's energy and feel old? With bioidentical hormone replacement, that youthful energy can return!

I have witnessed this in many patients, including myself. I found my energy declining in my 50's and blood work revealed my testosterone to be less than optimal. Since I started supplementation, I have had a return of my youthful energy and motivation! My results were so great, I decided to share them with my patients. In the last few years I have treated thousands of patients with testosterone, with equally great results! I have heard patients say that they haven't felt this good in 15 years. A typical internal medicine patient comes in with a laundry list of complaints. My Testosterone patients come in and say, "I feel great, keep doing what you are doing doc, because you have changed my life!" and might I add the complaint list is gone!

Estradiol also improves energy, especially in those severely deficient, as in menopause. IMO, it is not as potent an energizer as testosterone, but nonetheless it will move the meter strongly in the right direction. It can also make life changing effects.

So, is better energy really reversing the aging process? Well in this case, it certainly reverses the symptoms of aging, and for many people, just feeling younger is sufficient to satisfy then. These symptom improvements are more than just symptom relief. Studies show that testosterone improves the function of mitochondria. Mitochondria are the cell parts that produce 95% of your cells and bodies energy. You are making more energy, so it is no wonder that you feel more energetic!

Many scientists believe the mitochondrial theory of disease. Your body requires energy for all body functions. As mitochondrial function declines with age, the body has less energy to perform its normal body functions. As functions decline, disease develops. Improving mitochondrial function is key to preventing the disease process and testosterone improves it. Evidence is still preliminary for estradiol and mitochondrial function, but it appears favorable also.

There is a lot more evidence in the age reversal process. Most people associate failing memory to age. Both testosterone and estradiol improve brain function and memory. In fact, testosterone is known to stimulate the production of new brain cells! Age causes loss of brain cells, but testosterone and estradiol do the opposite. They make new brain cells Isn't that our fear? The fear of worsening mental function leading to dementia? These hormones can move the meter in the other direction to more brain cells and better function, the reverse of what the aging process does.

What about weight gain? With age, weight builds up in the middle. With testosterone (and other hormonal decline) weight builds up in the middle. If your bio identically replace testosterone, the abdominal weight gain reverses (given the proper environment of good diet and activity). SO, was it age that did it, or was it hormonal declines? I see improvements in belly fat even without dietary changes. Patients are gratified by the weight loss that occurs with replacement. Not only are they pleased with the number, but also with the weights distribution. Less belly fat makes a person appear healthier and younger. Well, in fact they are healthier! Getting rid of inflammatory belly fat is a positive for health and appearance. Testosterone improves muscle mass. Higher muscle mass is corelated with longer life and better health. More muscle definition also makes a person appear (and is) healthier, HRT (hormone replacement therapy) provides a healthier, and more attractive, youthful appearing body.

Estradiol has more of a neutral effect on weight. In fact, in large doses, it can cause weight gain. This may also depend on the method of administration. Estradiol by mouth, as in birth control pills or other estradiol preparations, is converted in the liver and can cause undesirable effects. It can cause weight gain when given by mouth, amongst other undesirable side effects. It can raise sugar craving, promote inflammation (which we know is bad) and increase diabetic tendencies. I avoid prescribing estradiol by mouth and I prescribe the right amounts when given by pellet, injection or cream.

So, what about bone density. With age, and the decline of hormones, bones soften in both men and women, leading to age related osteoporosis. But is it age or hormonal decline that is causing this condition? It turns out that if you replace the deficient hormones of testosterone and estradiol, new bone formation will occur, and the process begins to reverse! In fact, although medicine has concocted many treatment options for osteoporosis using chemical medicines, HRT is the most effective treatment by raising bone density about 10%. The bone produced is functional bone, in other words it is effective in preventing fractures because it is naturally produced. The "best medication" options raise bone density at best 6%. Worse, the type of bone produced does not have normal structure and is often ineffective for fracture prevention.

What about blood sugar metabolism? As people age their blood sugars will worsen, especially if they have a lot of abdominal obesity. Diabetes is often thought to be age related. Well, both testosterone and estradiol improve blood sugar metabolism. Diabetes risk is lowered 22% in those with optimal levels! So, they help prevent the disease of aging diabetes!

What about sexual function? As men and women age, they experience lower libido, atrophy (wasting) of the genital areas, and reduced ability to achieve orgasm. These symptoms of poorer libido and function can be reversed with optimal hormone replacement. Your calendar years may be high, but you don't have to lose your sexuality because of it. We can reverse that "age related" sexual decline with HRT!

What about cardiovascular illness? That is thought to be an age-related decline in function. Both testosterone and estradiol improve the function of the arteries and heart and therefore is helpful in the prevention of cardiovascular illness. Estradiol maintains the elasticity of arteries. Less illness is indicative of a healthier, more youthful body.

What about quality of life issues. Older people are supposed to be unhappier. The grumpy old man syndrome is related to hormone decline. The hot flashing explosive menopausal woman is related to hormone decline. If we fix the decline, all quality of life measures improves! Energy improves, mood improves, sleep improves, sex drive and function improve. Poor sleep is associated with aging. Isn't it awesome that we can improve these age-related symptoms with only 1 intervention?

What about wrinkles and aging skin? Estradiol specifically promotes more healthy, youthful appearing skin. Even your body appearance is more youthful.

What about muscle mass. Age causes a decline of muscle mass. This eventually causes problems with weakness, immobility and fall risk. These are signs of aging. Both testosterone and to some extent estradiol, improve muscle strength and function. You don't have to become that weak, frail, fall risk person. We can prevent that decline and reverse it!

But what if my doctor tells me my hormones are normal for my age?

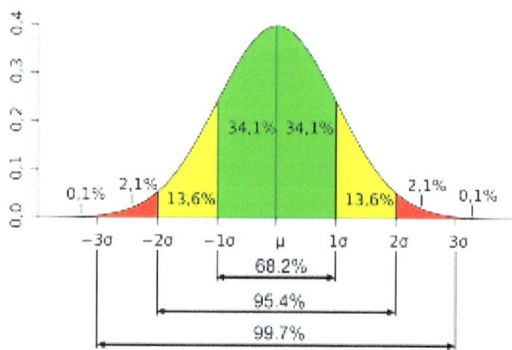

Well he probably will! The reason is most doctors practice like this. They determine normal values based on population averages. Have you looked at our population recently? Obesity is rampant! Overweight is everywhere. Do you want to be average in this unhealthy populations where 70% are overweight or obese? I certainly don't want average, but that is how conventional medicine practices.

Most doctors practice like this. If your result is in the lower 2% or upper 2%, it is considered abnormal, but if it is in the 96% in the middle, too bad for you! You can be in the lower percentiles and have fatigue, moodiness, sleep disturbance, poor libido and sexual function, and experiencing the "symptoms of aging" like weight gain, brain fog, weakening muscles and bones, and this is still considered normal! But I don't want normal for my patients, I want OPTIMAL. Optimal is in the higher end of the curve, and that is where people function best in terms of quality of life measures, like energy mood, sleep, and sex function, but also in terms of internal health like brain function, bone density, blood sugar metabolism, muscle strength, cardiovascular health etc.! SO, do you want normal or optimal numbers? For me the answer is clear, optimal!

But what about the dangers. Most people, (and even many doctors) get their medical information from the media. The media has not gone to medical school. Their job is to get attention. 95% of all media stories have a negative slant. They don't have to provide a balanced report, only one that sells

Testosterone and estradiol have both had their media flogging. The flogging was a result for controversial studies and inaccurate biases that create fear in people from doing the right things for their body. Let's review them

Testosterone has been reported to cause prostate cancer. This was based on a single patient study in 1947 that was poorly documented. The fact is, that very low testosterone is a strong risk factor for the most aggressive and lethal form of prostate cancer. If you fear taking testosterone because of this, you may be INCREASING your likelihood of getting prostate cancer by avoiding testosterone! In Europe, and experimentally in California they are using testosterone to treat prostate cancer! In 1 study, patients treated for over 20 years with testosterone therapy for over 20 years did not show an increase in prostate cancer. I am not saying we should willy nilly throw testosterone into every prostate cancer patient. I am saying that the old biases are flawed and that each patient needs to be individually assessed for the risks and benefits of treatment.

What about cardiovascular disease? Didn't the media accuse testosterone of contributing to it? Again, this is strongly media biased. The most criticized is the VA study. This study has been reprimanded by the medical community because of the flawed design, and flawed interpretation. On further review, the treated group had fewer cardiovascular events! The VA has refused to retract the study despite intense criticism. Does the public hear the outcry? No, they just hear the initial fear generating story. Does the media give a balanced report on it? No, there are hundreds of studies that show benefit to the function of arteries and the heart with testosterone therapy. The medias job, though, is not to provide a medical education to the patient, but just to sensationalize reports to draw attention. Testosterone is beneficial to the cardiovascular condition. It needs to be. If you want to reproduce (which is one of its main functions) you need to have well-functioning sex organs, but also a sound cardiovascular system that can support the intercourse process. That would be an ironic trick from God, to promote procreation with hormones and then to kill the organism by robbing it of the cardiovascular health needed to accomplish it. No testosterone improves these functions to make reproduction possible.

Testosterone has been shown to improve the function of the vascular lining (endothelium) This decline with age and testosterone reverses that decline. Estradiol has been shown to decrease blood vessel plaque formation. Plaque formation is considered a disease of aging. Both testosterone and estradiol have been shown to decrease blood pressure. Elevated blood pressure is mostly idiopathic (meaning we don't know the cause) but it's incidence increases greatly with age.

What about estradiol? Isn't that cancer causing? Again, some of this bias was media created. It relates way back to the WHT (women's heart trial), way back in 2000.At that time, a study using Prempro (horse estrogen plus chemically altered progesterone) showed poor results, with a questionable increase in breast cancer. Did the media report that there are many extensive studies that show the opposite? no increase in cancer? No that would not be shocking enough. They need to enlarge the negative and avoid the positive as this provide a more exciting controversial review. Did the medial tell you that after more time and review, almost all the negative findings have been reversed? Breast cancer wasn't increased. In fact, it was never the estradiol to begin with! It was always the chemically altered progesterone (so called progestins) that was the culprit all along. You can't play with mother nature. It likes things in their natural unaltered structure, and it reacts badly to fakes.

Estradiol has been shown to improve skin health and produces a more youthful appearance. It has been shown to decrease wrinkles. These are visible signs of aging. The aging process cause a loss of collagen in the skin. Estradiol increases the amount of collagen and water content in the skin, making it appear thicker and softer and therefore decrease wrinkles and visible aging.

And what about death? Isn't that the ultimate sign of aging? 4 major good studies have shown a decreased risk of death from all causes with testosterone treatment. Although I don't have survival prolonging effects documented for estradiol, there are many studies that show a reduced incidence of cardiovascular disease, osteoporosis and dementia, which are 3 of the major causes of death in women, so it is intuitive that death should be reduced with estradiol also.

Now that you are convinced of the anti-aging properties if testosterone and estradiol, how do you get them? Unfortunately for both, it is not by mouth. Both testosterone and estradiol are metabolized through the liver after oral administration. This undesirable metabolism alters its effect in the system. Estradiol by mouth promotes inflammation, sugar cravings, clotting potential, blood pressure, liver inflammation, and more.

Testosterone by mouth can cause serious liver disease, mood disturbance, edema and more, I don't' recommend administration that method.

Next option is creams, Creams are poorly absorbed, the skin is designed to be protective, not an absorption vehicle for medications. In many cases I do get see a very good levels or response form the creams, but it varies. There are diligent patents that do get a good response. This is something that requires the discipline to administer daily, and many patients are not that diligent. They need to be rubbed in, so it also requires some patience. For women the main alternative to a cream is a patch, but these only addresses estradiol, and not testosterone. The main downside, (besides ineffective levels in many) is that creams, (and lesser extent patches) are transmissible to children and sex partners. For me, small children around is a deal breaker as they can cause early puberty in them. That is very undesirable.

Now welcome to the best alternative, which is pellet therapy. In this office procedure, we numb up the area of the buttocks and insert rice like pellets that area pure testosterone or estradiol. There is excellent absorption and this method avoids the direct metabolism through the liver and minimizes those side effects. I get much better absorption, levels and response! This takes compliance out of the equation. They will slow release over 3-6 months and there is nothing required from the patient to do. It is the easy button to get a good response without the daily cream responsibility The last options are injectables, many men do well with this option. The downsides to it are that testosterone has a short ½ life, so weekly administration is generally necessary. Some people just aren't comfortable with injections. The short half-life means that some people can start to run low towards the end of the week. Compliance also becomes an issue for some. If you don't do the shots, you don't get the results. Some women even choose this method as it is more affordable than pellet therapy

Now side effects need to be discussed 1 to1, but the main ones I look for are with testosterone, acne, hair loss or hair growth, edema, or signs of high estradiol, its metabolite. These could include breast soreness or swelling, moodiness, and eventually prostate issues. One should be aware that testosterone replacement in males can have contraceptive effects. People with low T have lower fertility. Replacement rebalances internal production, so fertility can decline. This is discussed face to face.

For estradiol, brief menstrual bleed or edema. The majority don't get these, but on occasion. There are treatments that could minimize these effects if they occur. Overall most patients benefit with little or no side effects. The side effects are pale in comparison to the positive result in quality of life and health.

Chapter 7

NUTRITIONAL SUPPLEMENTS

Besides not poisoning ourselves with sugar or inflammation, and reversing some of the damage done with hormone optimization, what other anti-aging tools do we have? Nutritional supplements.

It would be great if we could get all our nutrients from food, but let's face it, food has changed in our lifetime. Our diets are carbohydrate rich, and our foods are robbed of many nutrients by processing, use of GMO foods, and agricultural techniques.

Sub-optimal nutrition, or shall we call it malnutrition is rampant, even in our overfeed American society! There are many critical nutrients that 80% or more of Americans are deficient in. Unfortunately, the majority are unaware of these deficiencies.

The situation is more complicated than that. There are innumerable supplements available. I hear about a new one every day. They all sound good. If you take them all you can spend your whole day taking supplements and they can overwhelm your food intake. How do you know which to take? Which have the most benefits? It requires a tremendous amount of research to sort out this tangled web. Only someone as crazy as me would put the time in. You can benefit from my hard research by reading this.

It's even more complicated than that. In addition to hundreds of supplements, there a hundreds of manufacturers. How do you decide who to buy from? That is a very complex issue. Supplements are not regulated by the FDA, there is no quality control, you don't really know what you are getting in many cases. I have no more information than you regarding what is in these products. It's a little bit of a gamble if they have what they say.

So how do you decide? If you are hell bent on getting what you want, then I would go with the more reputable manufacturers like life extension or Mercola. There is still no guarantee, but I think the likelihood of getting what you are paying for is greater. The downside to this is that you must pay up for the quality, sometimes greatly! I take a ton of supplements. If I pay up for all of them, I will have to cut out about ½ of them for expense reasons. For that reason, I often utilize price as my guide and take my chances. If you are a purist, or only take few supplements, or are much wealthier than me, you may choose to pay up for quality. It's a personal decision.

I am going to rank the nutrients by documented health benefits. The gold standard for a supplement is if it prevented or reversed disease so well that it is documented to have life prolonging effects. I will grade these supplements an A. A second and desirable result would be to reduce the incidence of a major disease, but without documented life prolonging effects. I will rate these supplements a B. The last class is for supplement that don't have documented longevity benefits, nor clear cut disease protection, but are known to improve the underlying physiology that will promote a disease process. Those supplement, I will rate a C. I will also give a C if they improve quality of life issues like energy, mood and sleep.

So, for example, If I am talking about cardiovascular disease, lowering the death rate from it ranks A, lowering the incidence of new heart attacks second ranks B, and improving the blood vessel function, or reducing things like inflammation or sugar that contribute to it would rank C.

So, can you guess the number 1 nutrient? I give you some choices. Multivitamin, Magnesium, Omega 3, or Vitamin D? Which is most effective?

If you guessed Vitamin D, you are much smarter than the average bear. Most would choose a multivitamin, which is Buzz, INCORRECT!

Why vitamin D? 80% or more are deficient even in Florida. There are no good dietary sources. Milk provides 100 IU, whereas you need 5,000 IU daily, you would have to drink 50 glasses of milk daily! I do not recommend that. A multivitamin contains only 400 IU. You would have to take 12 to get the right dosage.

What does it do? Well everything. It is the #1 most beneficial nutrient. It is useful for weight control, people with low levels cannot lose weight. It decreases diabetes risk in ½ and pre-diabetes by 91%! People with low levels have a 20 X risk of Alzheimer's! People with severe deficiency have a 71% higher risk of death. Deficiency leads to a 40% higher risk of cancer.

There are many other benefits. It improves mood. Vitamin D is as effective as standard anti-depressant therapy! It improves general achiness. It decreases back pain by 50%! It improves immune function a blood pressure control, in short, if you can only take 1 supplement, take this one. It wins hands down for disease prevention, longevity, and quality of life issues.

What about Vitamin D toxicity? This is the most overblown risk ever! There have been very few cases worldwide. You must seriously overdose for prolonged time periods to get this. Yet, many people are aware of this and are afraid to take it, or afraid to take anything but a miniscule dose because of it. American labs signal reading over 100 as toxic. Research from the middle east show that many patients there have reading in the 100-150 area with no ill effects. Despite its rarity, I still recommend checking levels every 6 months or so, especially in those on high doses, but also for others. Many patients complete their bottle and forget to renew so those not taking Vitamin D are at far greater risk than those taking too much. Most outlets don't sell anything over 10,000 IU, and often sell supplements with as little as 400 IU,1000 IU, or 2,000 IU. These doses are way too low to achieve optimal levels, an optimal level is in the 50-70 level, really 70 is best. I personally must take 20,000 IU daily to achieve that and I have many other patients taking 15-20,000 IU WHILE THEY ARE MONITORED with levels.

Recommend dose is tremendously variable. In general, I recommend a starting does of 5,000 IU. This may vary some. If you have advanced liver or kidney disease, consult your physician on dosing. If you are a frail old lady, you may require less. Many people do require more, but I recommend that based on levels. The easier, and more effective button is to take the 50,000 IU D3 weekly off amazon. Your Physician Might want to prescribe Vitamin D2 instead. I don't recommend that. D3 is the bodies preferred form, and some studies suggested a higher death rate with D2, you can get D3 more easily and at a better price than D2 anyway.

I will be giving you some ideas of price. For reference I am using Amazon prices, which is where I get most of mine I use them because of greater choices, better prices and convenience. I hear daily patients tell me that they ran out 2 months ago and have not made it back to their health food store yet. Amazon is the easy button to avoid these lapses. 1 click and it's there tomorrow, with the best price. I will put in expected monthly cost. In most cases I am buying a minimum of 60-90 days' worth, so the price will be divided to represent what the monthly cost will be even though I am getting 3 months at a time.

Vitamin D3 5,000 IU (no specific brand) $1-4 monthly or Rating A

Vitamin D3 50,000 IU weekly Biotec $1.50 monthly

Ok, so if you can only take 1 supplement, Vitamin D 3 is the clear winner. Vitamin D 3 gets an A rating!

Now for second place. It's a close call, but Omega 3 wins out.
Omega 3 is an essential nutrient. If you don't supply your body with it, you will be deficient, it can't make it. Omega 3 's are critical for brain function. It is an essential part for brain structure. It can also induce new brain cells. Some studies suggest that it lowers risk of Alzheimer's by 31%!

It also reduces inflammation and therefore reduces cardiovascular

DR RAYMOND D. ADAMCIK

disease by about 10%, I t reduces overall death by 8%, It improves triglycerides and "good cholesterol" HDL and more. If you are a big eater of tuna, salmon, sardines, mackerel or anchovies, your intake may be such that you need less than the recommended amount below.

Krill oil is another alternative. It is better absorbed so some people can get by with a lower dosage, especially if they already eat some fish. It also contains choline, which is brain food and astaxanthin which is a powerful anti-oxidant. Downsides are its higher cost, especially if more than 1 gram is required daily.

Omega 3 (fish oil) 2 grams daily (no specific manufacturer) $4-9 monthly Rating A

Or Krill oil 1 gram daily $10 monthly

What about mercury? Mercury poisoning is overdone. I am sure there are some cases out there, I have yet to see one. However, I see patients with insufficient intake of this essential nutrient daily. If you are deficient, you are certain to have health consequences. I take the risk that I may get a rare toxicity to correct the certain deficiency and certain health consequences in its absence. I see many patients depriving themselves of this essential nutrient to prevent an extremely rare condition. Life is an experiment. Leaving the house, or crossing the street is a risk. We can't be paralyzed in life for fear of ever taking a risk. We all must assess the potential benefits versus the risk for every action. In the case the benefit is certain and the risk infinitesimal. I take fish oil and lose no sleep over it. If you are a worrier, then this is one circumstance that you might consider paying up for a Mercola or Life Extension brand.

Magnesium Threonate 500 mg (No specific manufacturer) or Magnesium Citrate or Glycinate $6.00 Monthly Rating A

Next is magnesium. 80% are deficient in magnesium, Magnesium used to be present in foods, but soil depletion has limited its availability even in those that consume magnesium rich foods. Magnesium is critical for energy production. In addition to helping fatigue it also helps sleep and mood.

Magnesium's critical for heart rhythm stabilization, and for blood pressure control, it decreases risk for elevated blood pressure. It improves blood sugar control and decreases diabetes risk. It also decreases cardiovascular risk and people with higher magnesium intakes are 9% less likely to die!

Magnesium Threonate can get to the brain so it is useful for brain fog. Citrate and Glycinate are well absorbed and less expensive alternative. Magnesium Oxide is poorly absorbed, but helps better for constipation

These 3 nutrients are the cornerstone to replacing the critical deficiencies. These will have the highest impact on your health but short term and long term and are most applicable to everyone. They certainly aren't the only nutrients I recommend. Additional nutrients are more patient specific and more optionable

Vitamin K is the next deficiency, I recommend

Super K by life extension $7 monthly Rating A

Vitamin K1 and K2. They help protect against 4 major illness. Cancer, diabetes, osteoporosis and cardiovascular disease. The numbers are quite impressive About 80% of patients are Vitamin K deficient. There are 2 main forms,

K1 decreases death by 36%, cancer 46% metabolic syndrome, Coronary heart disease by 21% and diabetes 17%-51% (depending on dose) and metabolic syndrome (pre-diabetes) by 27%-82%. Higher levels if the patient is closer to the diagnosis already

K2 decreased death by 26%, cancer death 28%, prostate cancer death 63%, coronary heart disease death 57%, and diabetes risk 7%
You may not feel much from vitamin k immediately, but your health will reward you on down the road. It's an optional nutrient for those that don't care how long you live, but otherwise if you are a decent supplement taker I strongly recommend it.

Then next optional nutrient is vitamin C

Vitamin C 1,000 mg (or more) daily (no specific manufacturer) $2 monthly Rating A

Many studied now document the effectiveness of Vitamin C to improve immunity. It is also an anti-oxidant, and studies suggest cardiovascular protection from its action. Lower levels of Vitamin C have a 57% higher mortality. And a 62 % higher risk of cancer deaths. Cardiovascular death is reduced 42% in men and 25% in women with high dose therapy!! Part of its mechanism is to protect "bad cholesterol" from oxidation (inflammatory damage). Vitamin C reduces LDL cholesterol from being oxidized by 75%! You can't get this from other sources you would have to eat 17 oranges a day or take 10 multi-vitamins to get this dosage, hence it is listed separately.

The next 4 are more optional nutrients. These involve the function of the mitochondria. The mitochondria are parts of the cell that make 95% of the cells and the bodies energy. Energy is required to perform all body functions. There is a mitochondrial theory if disease that says that their functional decline is responsible for ALL diseases! If you improve mitochondrial function, it could help energy and improve metabolism, and therefor improves weight control also. If you want to improve general health, energy, or weight control, you may choose one or more of these supplements.

Carnitine 2000 mg daily $7monthly Rating B

Carnitine promotes the shuttle of fat across the mitochondrial border to be burned so it stimulates the burning of belly fat, but also improves muscle mass and brain function! That's a triple play. It promotes weight loss, improves memory improves heart function and decreases the death rate in heart patients. It improves muscle strength performance, stamina, and fatigue. It also reduces inflammation, lower triglycerides and more! Although this is optional, there are many reasons to take it.

Green tea extract $2 monthly Rating A

Do you drink large quantities of coffee or green tea? If so, you may not need this supplement. Both coffee and green tea are metabolic stimulants that promote weight loss, reduce diabetes risk, reduces Alzheimer's and Parkinson's risk and prolongs life. Green tea also decreases cancer risk. It has been shown to decrease coronary artery disease by 64%, and stroke by 32%, It has been shown to decrease the progression of prostate cancer by 90%! The extract has equal to 17 cups of green teas active component ECGC (without the caffeine component) This supplement is most useful for those that want better energy and weight, but its health benefits are so broad, anyone could benefit from it.

Ubiquinol 100 mg daily (Jarrow seems to have the best price) $8 monthly Rating B

Ubiquinol is the active form co coenzyme Q10. You must take twice as much of co-q10 to get an equivalent dosage, but it is inactive, and it requires a youthful energetic metabolism to activate, hence I recommend the active form.

Ubiquinol improves heart function, slows the atherosclerotic process, lowers the death rate in heart patients by 50%! It also lowers blood pressure by 12/6, improves blood sugar control, reduces inflammation, improves physical performance and prolongs life in some species.

Again, this supplement has diffuse and important health benefits. Tired and overweight patients will benefit best, but all could potentially see long term benefits.

Mitochondrial energy optimizer with PQQ (life extension only)
$12 monthly Rating C

This supplement contains many ingredients that are essential for good mitochondrial function including PQQ which gives you more mitochondria to make more energy. It most helpful for fatigued people that want to promote weight loss, but as mitochondrial function is critical for all body functions, it should have similar general health and disease protective qualities.

Life extension 2 per day capsules $6 monthly

Multivitamins are the most commonly taken nutritional supplement. Many patients think that their diet can provide most of the nutrition needed and the multivitamin can fill in the rest. They are in denial that they can obtain all their essential nutrients from 1 tablet. They also overestimate the value of their diet because

#1 Some nutrients are present in food in only trace amounts, and unfortunately the same one's lacking in multivitamins. Examples would include critical Vitamin D, magnesium, omega 3, vitamin K, Vitamin C, and micronutrient minerals. If you don't take these nutrients separately, you will be deficient in them like 80% of our population

#2 Most are not eating the diet that gives them essential minerals and vitamins. Are you getting your 5 fruit and vegetable servings daily? Do you eat fatty fish like salmon or tuna 2 x weekly?

#3 Many people are nutrient depleted because they eat high

carbohydrate foods that deplete vitamins,

#4 Most people cook their food that destroys ½ of the nutrients.

#5Food isn't what it used to be. they are GMO modified foods, often full of pesticides, and hormonally altered

So, food can be not only nonnutritive, but also toxic!

Besides eating correctly, multivitamins in general are a poor solution to malnutrition. Despite all the dietary limitations, less than 1 % are critically deficient in the common vitamins not mentioned above.

There have been several studies of multivitamins and none this far have proven to be effective for preventing disease or death. In fact, on some occasions the studies have shown them to be detrimental.

Why this contradiction between the logical administration of nutrients and unimpressive response? Part of the problem is the most essential vitamins are not present in the right quantities nor in the right form to achieve the desired benefits. Examples would be vitamin D (which is not a vitamin but a hormone) is usually only present in 400 IU when in fact, 5000 IU is necessary for good health. Vitamin E is present in its least effective form. Vitamin K, (which is quite important) is usually absent. Vitamin C is useful, but in much larger amounts than those in a multivitamin, and the same for many B Vitamins.

If you still want to take multivitamin, I only recommend 1,

Life extension 2 per day capsules. Rating C

I have compared them to many others that fall short. It contains the right amount of the right vitamins in the right form, with bonus micromineral contents and other nutrients. There is evidence that the B vitamins provide some quality of life improvements like mood improvement, brain function, and energy productions, which gives it the C rating, as longevity and clear-cut disease prevention are undocumented.

I recommend this Behind correcting the more critical deficiencies discussed above.

Are these the only nutrients I recommend? No, but many of the others are on an individual basis depending on each patient's symptoms, conditions, and willingness to take preventative supplements. The next ones will be somewhat in order of preference.

The other caveat to my ranking is that practically no one wants to put in the millions of dollars to conduct a trail on a supplement that anyone can make without a patent. There are many supplements further on my list that have tremendous effects on physiologic parameters, but no one has done outcome studies on them. An example of this might be astaxanthin, which shows the physiologic properties that could prevent many illnesses, maybe better than the higher up supplements, but there are no documented trials yet to prove its effectiveness. That being said here are some more supplements I recommend to selected patients in order of effectiveness

Olive oil! Rating B Technically you could say this is not a supplement, it's a food. Well yes, it is, but I take it as a supplement. It's on the list because it reduces cardiovascular disease by as much as 44%. It also improves the function of blood vessel lining (endothelium). It raises good cholesterol (HDL) and reduces the damage to bad cholesterol (LDL) and its levels. I add it to my foods, like salads. You can also use it for cooking, but coconut oil is slightly better for cooking. 1 tablespoon a day is all it takes.

Next is Vitamin E, but not just regular vitamin E, it must contain Vitamin E tocotrienols. Vitamin E has 8 forms. Most people who take a supplement take alpha tocopherols. This is the most common, and the one most patients take. It is the one that was included in clinical studies. The problem with this one is that it appears to be the least effective of the vitamin e forms and can block the effects of the more potent ones. Therefore, some of the studies on Vitamin E have been negative showing possible harm! For this reason, I don't recommend generic Vitamin E. I prefer the supplements that contain all the active forms, especially the 4 tocotrienol forms. Life extension multi contains only 4/8 forms. That is way better than most, and it still misses the 4 most active forms.

Toco-sorb, doctors best tocotrienols and Life extension tocotrienols are brands I have used Rating C

The overall results are quite good. In Alzheimer's disease it reduced plaques 64%(plaques though to be intimately involved in disease progression). It improves heart muscle function. It Lowers so called "bad cholesterol "42%. It stabilizes artery plaque. It reduces inflammation. It improves blood sugar control and insulin sensitivity. It may have cancer protective effect and improves fatty liver. Overall it has diffuse helpful effects, but specific mortality or disease prevention data is sparse.

Pomegranate (no specific manufacturer) Rating C

49

There is plenty of evidence that it improves the physiology that causes cardiovascular disease, but no hard evidence on mortality or incidence of cardiovascular disease. It has been shown to decrease the thickness of plaque by about 30% It decreases damaged (oxidized) LDL (bad) cholesterol by 90%! It also lowers Blood pressure by 12%, lowers triglycerides and raises good cholesterol 5 %. These all suggest a lower incidence of cardiovascular disease and death would be likely, but not confirmed by any studies. I recommend it in higher cardiovascular risk patients.

Selenium 200 mg (no specific manufacturer) Rating B

Selenium deficiency is common, and it is an important nutrient. If you take the life extension 2 per day, you can skip this one. Selenium is critically involved in cancer protection. There is a 37% decreased risk of any cancer with it, and a 63% lower risk of prostate cancer with it.

Besides cancer protection it is also necessary for thyroid function. It is a powerful anti-oxidant, improves immunity, and decreases heart disease risk. Its' and optional nutrient important for cancer protection, and better taken as part of the life extension multivitamin.

Zinc (50 mg) (any manufacturer) Rating B

Zinc has proven benefits in shortening the course and frequency pf respiratory infection. It also reduces diabetes risk 10% and lowers central obesity 12%. Life extension 2 daily has 25 mg. If you have a respiratory illness, or want better protection, then consider adding this especially during acute infections

Astaxanthin 4 mg (no specific manufacturer) Rating C

Astaxanthin is a very powerful anti-oxidant. It is 64 times more potent than vitamin C! If its anti-inflammatory effects translate over to disease protection, it should be amazing, but there are no clinical trials to document that. It does reduce inflammation, enhances heart health and does reduce stroke risk. It improves brain function, combats cancer, boosts immunity, improves blood sugar control, and activates a longevity gene. These are all great theoretical reasons to take it, but full-blown disease protection and longevity benefits are not documented YET. It may be a magic yet untested weapon. It is present in krill oil, so you may not require this supplement if you are already taking krill oil. There are many diffuse physiologic benefits to this and I recommend it to those who want to aggressively decrease their disease risk with supplements.

Taurine 3000 mg (no specific manufacturer) Rating C

This is one of my favorite nutrients due to its many favorable physiologic effects, but longevity and disease protection are not clearly documented.

Taurine is an amino acid. Its actions are predominately on the neurologic system and cardiovascular but has effects elsewhere too.

In the brain it reduces the inflammatory process associated with Alzheimer's disease and Parkinson's disease. It protects brain cells and mitochondria from damage and dysfunction. It promotes the formation of new brain cells. It improves cognition and recall. It is also helpful for neuropathy and helps provide their covering and induces new nerve growth.

It has other beneficial properties. People deficient in it have higher cardiovascular risk, Treatment improves arterial stiffness, heart function, and exercise time. It reduces insulins resistance and improves metabolic syndrome, it reduces risk of hypertension 22%. It reduces inflammation 29%

Deficiency has a 184% higher risk of obesity! It improves fat metabolism and increases muscle mass. There are no studies to show that supplementation reverses this risk.

NAD+ 50-100 mg (prefer life extension but other options acceptable) Rating C

The anti-aging medical community has recently gotten very excited about it's potential. NAD is found in every cell. It's an activated form of niacin that is not present in multivitamins. Its function is to transfer energy and it turns off genes that accelerate the aging process! Because of this property it has been reported to increase lifespan in some species. A decline of this nutrient causes degeneration of the nervous system, increase fat storage in the belly and liver, resistance to insulin, fatigue and muscle weakness. Treatment improves endurance and memory. It promotes weight loss and increases your mitochondrial number. This is another supplement that the physiology looks great, but definitive studies to show improvements in longevity in humans and disease reduction is sparse. I recommended for those that want to aggressively supplements to stave of aging and disease.

Alpha Lipoic acid 1200 mg (no specific manufacturer) Rating C

Alpha lipoic acid is a critical co-factor in energy production. It helps regenerate the master anti-oxidant glutathione. It is also an antioxidant and reduces inflammation. It improves diabetes associated neuropathy pain. It's been shown to reduce mental decline in Alzheimer's disease. I recommend it as a supplement in those with Alzheimer's, diabetic neuropathy or those wanting an aggressive approach to improving their metabolism.

Blueberry extract (no specific manufacturer) Rating C

Blueberries have amazing effects! You can eat blueberries as I did, but the expense, especially in off season is very high and it is difficult to do long term.

There has been extensive work in animal and fireflies that confirm life extension 28-35%! That is a huge number.

Besides prolonging life in animals, it has been shown to improve memory and cognitive abilities.

Other effects are multiple It stimulates fat and sugar burning and improves the metabolic syndrome by improving insulin resistance, it reduces oxidation, reduces arterial stiffness.

It is an aggressive supplement to add but should be considered because of the possible life prolonging effects and more.

Quercetin 500 mg (no specific manufacturer) Rating C

Quercetin has multiple beneficial physiologic effects for the heart, it triggers plaque regression. It improves the function of the vessel lining (endothelium) It lowers cardiovascular risk and improves exercise tolerance by 13%. It improves insulin sensitivity and reduces blood pressure.

It reduces inflammation and aids in the production of the master anti-oxidant glutathione. This leads to neuroprotective effects and may be helpful for preventing Alzheimer's disease and Parkinson's diseases.

It decreases fatty liver, and promote weight loss through loss of belly fat

Overall these are helpful, especially for cardiovascular health or for general health as an aggressive add on nutrient.

Resveratrol 20 mg (no specific manufacturer) Rating C

Resveratrol is derived from red wine and may be partially responsible for the French paradox. (low cardiac risk with what was thought to be a bad diet, now debatable if the butter rich diet was bad). It takes 220 glasses if red wine to get 20 mg of resveratrol.

It prolongs life in animals that show less deterioration of their muscles and nervous system. It activates a gene (sirt1) which slows the aging process As far as the neurologic system, it improves brain flow, suppresses brain inflammation, and may improve memory and learning.

It's helpful for the vascular system. It reduces vascular stiffness, reduces blood pressures, and raises good cholesterol(HDL) Its shown to improve blood sugar, and improve insulin sensitivity.

It has cancer protective properties. It improves fat metabolism.

There are animal studies and physiologic studies that support it, but human studies showing longevity or disease prevention are lacking in substance.

Sam-e 400-800 mg (no specific manufacturer) Rating C

Sam-e helps to recycle neuro-transmitters and is therefore helpful in depression. It has been shown in clinical trials to be of benefit.
It is important in the synthesis of the master anti-oxidant glutathione. It helps repair DNA so prevents cell death.

It is useful in osteoarthritis by stimulating cartilage production. That gives it potential reversal technology.

It is depleted in Alzheimer's and Parkinson's disease and thought useful in fibromyalgia and colitis.

Turmeric (also known as curcumin) 1000-2000 mg (no specific manufacturer) Rating B

Many of my patients take turmeric and swear by it. It is most known for its anti-inflammatory properties and has been shown superior to traditional anti-inflammatories in the treatment of arthritis without the high side effect profile that traditional anti-inflammatories have. (up to 53% high incidence if stroke, GI bleeding, liver abnormalities, etc.)

It had many other purported benefits. It improves the immune system, has cancer fighting abilities, and prolongs life in some species! It improves the production of new mitochondria and hence energy production.

It has theoretical advantages in Alzheimer's disease and Parkinson's disease by its actions of triggering proteins.

It has been shown to perform as well as traditional anti-depressants in 1 controlled study and can be combines with them for even greater response.

NAC 1200 mg (no specific manufacturer) Rating C

N -acetyl Cysteine is the critical nutrient needed to produce the master anti-oxidant Glutathione. Through this reaction it regulates inflammation. It helps detox the liver and improves insulin sensitivity.

It is most useful in those with rampant inflammation or liver function abnormalities.

PQQ 20 mg (available through life extension and in mitochondrial energizer but can be take separately) Rating C

This largely unheard if nutrient is an essential nutrient and had been labeled vitamin b13 at one point.

It stimulates the formation of new mitochondria and therefore energy production. It reduces inflammation.

It's helpful in the neurologic system by stimulating the formation of new nerve cells, improving memory, and improves walking in Parkinson's disease. It may protect against neurologic damage of Alzheimer's.

Probiotic 10 25 billion (now manufacturer) Rating C

Probiotics are a cutting-edge treatment. I have been to whole weekend conferences largely dedicated to them. I cannot present all the data here.

In general, there is no question that internal bacteria contribute, or at the root of many if not most of medical issues. They have been clearly linked to obesity, diabetes, coronary disease, depression, colon cancer, Alzheimer's, autism, fibromyalgia multiple sclerosis, and more.

Studies are sparse, some have shown effectiveness in mood disorders, but others show the potential for physiologic improvements.

There are many problems with probiotics. Number 1 is that many don't survive stomach acid. There are trillions of internal bacteria, so many supplements (like yogurt) that contain 1 million is a tiny drop in the bucket. The dose is too small to have an effect Many probiotics are already inactivated before you take them.

There are some specific bacteria that are thought to trigger disease and some that are rumored effective against certain disease. The proof is slim, however. I have not seen any good studies to show that a specific probiotic was able to alter the physiology enough to document an improvement in longevity or disease incidence. This field is in its infancy right now. Your choice may vary on your condition, Pro-10 has a very large number of probably useful bacteria that are coated to escape the stomach acid destruction.

Xanthohumol 2 caps sold as hops flowers (nature's way) Rating C

Xanthohumol is derived from hops flowers. It has been shown to promote weight loss. It promotes new mitochondria.

It also lowers blood sugar and improves insulin sensitivity. It lowers triglycerides.

It reduces inflammation is an anti-oxidant and theorized helpful in brain, joint, and cardiovascular health.

Melatonin 10-20 mg (no specific manufacturer) Rating B

Melatonin triggers the onset of sleep. Besides that, it has many other functions. It improves blood sugar metabolism. It relaxes muscles and nerves during sleep. It helps remove toxins, improves mood, improves immune system, and improves mitochondrial function. It stimulates growth hormone and thyroid hormone. There is evidence that is cancer protective for breast and prostate cancers. There is good evident that it is helpful for prevention of Alzheimer's and Parkinson's disease.

Deficiencies are linked to obesity, cardiovascular disease, osteoporosis and depression.

Symptoms of deficiency include nervousness, onset insomnia fatigue, morning sleepiness irritability, etc.

L-theanine 200 mg (no specific manufacturer) Rating C

L-theanine is an amino acid found in green tea, it has calming effects by blocking glutamate and increasing GABA (the calming neurotransmitter) It can improve alertness and prevents blood pressure surges under stress. It improves function of the endothelium (blood vessel lining)

MCT oil (no specific manufacturer) Rating C

MCT is a supplement that can be bought online or at your local health food store. It is derived, from coconuts or palm kernel oil or butter. It can be absorbed directly through the intestinal wall. The brain can metabolize it and it improves brain and neurologic function. It suppresses appetite and promotes weight loss. It has also been shown improve energy and athletic performance. It improves fatty liver. It reduces the risk heart disease, diabetes, cancer, and auto-immune disease. I add it to my coffee in the AM

L-glutamine 2-5,000 mg (no specific manufacturer) Rating C

L-glutamine is an essential amino acid. It stimulates growth hormone and improves metabolism, fat burning and muscle growth. It is also very useful for anyone with Gastro-intestinal disease as it helps heal the lining of the intestine. It is very useful in leaky gut, Crohns disease, auto-immune disorders and other GI disorders.

Condition specific nutrients

In this section, I will summarize my favorite nutrients for specific organ problems. In some cases, the full list could be quite long, but I will only list my top 5

Cancer fighting nutrients

Vitamin D 3

Vitamin k1, and k2

Selenium

Energy nutrients

Magnesium

Ubiquinol

Alpha lipoic acid

Carnitine

d-ribose

Life extension multin2 daily (b vitamins)

Weight loss nutrients

Green tea extract

Carnitine

Ubiquinol

Vitamin D

Vitamin C 3,000 mg

Heart Nutrients

Ubiquinol

Omega 3

Vitamin k2

Green tea extract

Pomegranate

Raise HDL (good cholesterol)

Carnitine

Ubiquinol

Magnesium

Resveratrol

Neuropathy

Taurine

Alpha lipoic acid

Glutathione or NAC

Osteoporosis

Vitamin d3

Magnesium

Calcium aspartate 800 mg

Vitamin k2

HRT

Mood disorders

Vitamin d3

Life extension 2 daily (b vitamins)

Zinc

Sam-e

Glutathione

GABA

Probiotics

Omega 3

Liver nutrients

Chlorophyllin

NAC (or glutathione)

Milk thistle

DIM

Improve GI system

Probiotics

Berberine

Glutamine 5000 mg

Improve Neurotransmitters

Omega 3

5 HTP up to 2000 mg

Sam-e

Best anti-aging nutrients

NAC

Gamma tocotrienol (vitamin e tocotrienols)

ECGC (green tea extract)

Diabetes supplements

Chromium

Alpha lipoic acid

Magnesium

Carnitine

Berberine

Carnosine

Taurine

quercetin

Life prolonging nutrients

Vitamin D

Omega 3

Magnesium

Vitamin C

Brain nutrients

Vitamin D

Omega 3

Magnesium threonate

Blueberries

Taurine

Inflammation

Ubiquinol

Green tea

Omega 3

Quercetin

Vitamin d

So, add the essential nutrients that will assist in longevity, disease prevention, and optimal body functions.

Chapter 8

PHYTONUTRIENTS

So, we need the right food categories, the right hormones, the right supplements, now for the finer points of the diet. This is an optional complicated segment. If you are not too interested in technicalities you may skip to the chapter end summary.

Now that we know how to avoid the toxicity of food, how do we improve the nutrition of food? The answer by making sure they have phytonutrients.

The term "Phyto" originated from a Greek word meaning plant. Phytonutrients are certain organic components of plants, and these components are thought to promote human health. Fruits, vegetables, grains, legumes, nuts and teas are rich sources of phytonutrients. Unlike the traditional nutrients (protein, fat, vitamins, minerals), phytonutrients are not "essential" for life.

Phytonutrients may:

- Serve as antioxidants
- Enhance immune response
- Enhance cell-to-cell communication
- Alter estrogen metabolism
- Convert to vitamin A (beta-carotene is metabolized to vitamin A)
- Cause cancer cells to die (apoptosis)
- Repair DNA damage caused by smoking and other toxic exposures
- Detoxify carcinogens through the activation of the cytochrome

P450 and Phase II enzyme systems
- Enhance weight loss
- Improve bone density
- Lower blood pressure and cardiovascular risk
- Improve blood sugar and insulin metabolism
- Improve brain function

How you get these amazing nutrients? Short answer? Vegetables and Fruits. So how are we at getting in these nutrients? Not good at all.

Only 49% get an average of 3 vegetable servings per day (3 minimum number). However, dark green vegetables and deep yellow vegetables each represent only 0.2 daily servings.

On any given day about 29% of the population consumes at least the minimum number of servings of fruit recommended (2 servings per day)

Fruit and vegetable consumption has been linked to decreased risk of stroke -- both hemorrhagic and ischemic stroke. Each increment of three daily servings of fruits and vegetables equated to a 22% decrease in risk of stroke, including transient ischemic attack.

Averaging more than 2 servings of Dark green and yellow vegetables had 46% less heart disease and 76 % less cancer compared to those that had less than 1 serving daily.

Fruits and vegetables are the largest source of phytonutrients. There are many classes of phytonutrients. The best-known phytonutrients are the carotenoids, flavonoids, polyphenols, indoles, lingams and isoflavones.

Let's start with my favorite the flavonoids.

Flavonoids

There are more than 6,000 unique flavonoids, each has its own health benefit. High flavonoid intake lowered heart disease 30% in some studies They are famous for antioxidant and anti-inflammatory effects. They also help with detoxifying the body, lower the risk of many chronic illnesses, and minimize weight gain with age. A recent study verified that those with the highest flavonoid intake had the least weight gain. These are found predominately in fruits and vegetables.

My favorite of the flavonoids is the anthocyanins.

Purple red fruit that contains anthocyanins. They were found to boost short term memory 100% and stimulate fat burning: Anthocyanins are found in dark purple or red grapes, cherries, and berries, including blueberries, blackberries, raspberries. The great bonus is that these fruits are low in sugar content too.

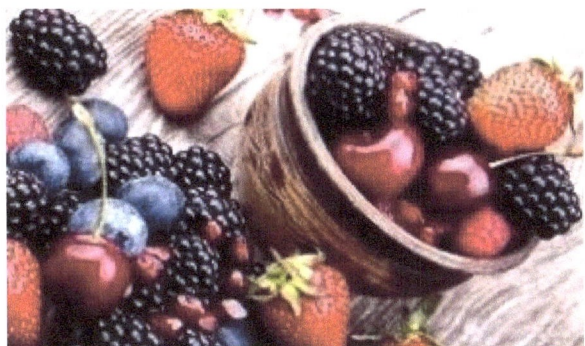

Figure 6-1 Purple and red fruit with anthocyanins

These flavonoids protect against oxidation, and the resultant free radicals' formation (prevents aging) which is thought to be at the root of chronic diseases (such as arthritis, atherosclerosis, diabetes and cancer) and to signs of aging, such as the loss of skin elasticity and cognitive function. Anthocyanidins have been found to have some unique features. Their free radical scavenging capabilities are thought to be more potent than many of the currently well-known vitamin antioxidants; anthocyanidins are estimated to have fifty times the antioxidant activity of both vitamin C and vitamin E!

Anthocyanins have been shown to have benefits beyond anti-oxidant activity, improved memory and promoting weight loss. Higher intake improves insulin resistance and lower inflammation! They have also been shown to improve blood sugar and blood pressure. They have been shown to lower heart disease risk! They improve the function of blood vessel linings (endothelium) and dysfunction of these can result in heart disease and ED. Guess what, they also decrease incidence of ED! So, if woody is your friend, feed him anthocyanins!

Quercetin is another flavonoid that has unique properties It has anti-inflammatory properties, is an antioxidant, and has been found to reduce blood pressure and lower LDL cholesterol. They also have cancer protective effects and may help fight chronic disease. It is associated with reduced risk of cardiovascular disease, blood pressure, and risk of certain cancers including lung, breast, colon, prostate, ovarian and endometrial cancer. Quercetin is found in green tea, red onion, broccoli, garlic, and green leafy vegetables.

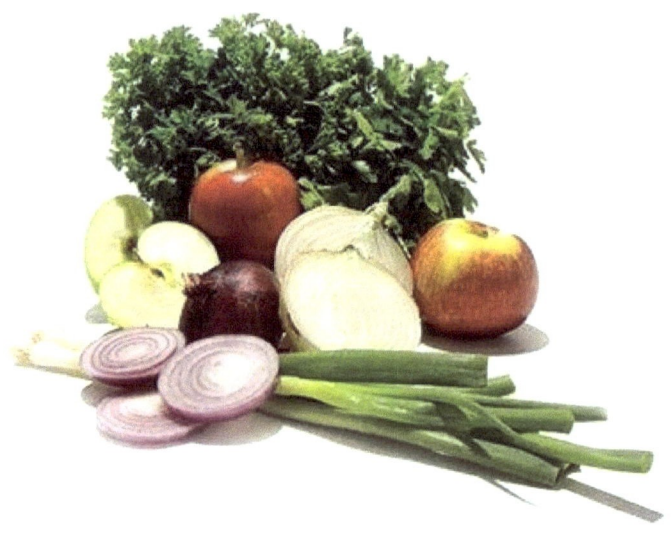

Figure 6-2 Quercetin sources

Vinegar is another source of flavonoids including catechin, and epicatechin (2 of my favorites) 1 tablespoon before meals has been shown to have beneficial effects, including reduced appetite and improved weight loss, improvements in blood sugar control, and at least in animals, improved blood pressure and cardiovascular effects.

Apigenin is a flavonoid found in herbs like parsley, thyme, chamomile, and in addition other foods like celery, Chinese cabbage, bell peppers, garlic and guava.

This class appears to promote the development of nerve cells. Although not yet proven in humans, animal studies suggest these foods could improve memory and overall brain function. Animal studies also suggest cancer protective effects. In human's chamomile tea was found to reduce thyroid cancer risk 80%.

Value	Per	Nutrient	Food
13506.20 mg	100 grams	Apigenin	Spices, parsley, dried
302.00 mg	100 grams	Apigenin	Parsley, raw
8.71 mg	100 grams	Apigenin	Peppermint, fresh
5.00 mg	100 grams	Apigenin	Thyme, fresh
4.61 mg	100 grams	Apigenin	Celery, raw
3.85 mg	100 grams	Apigenin	Rutabagas, raw
2.41 mg	100 grams	Apigenin	Celeriac, raw

Figure 6-3 apigenin sources

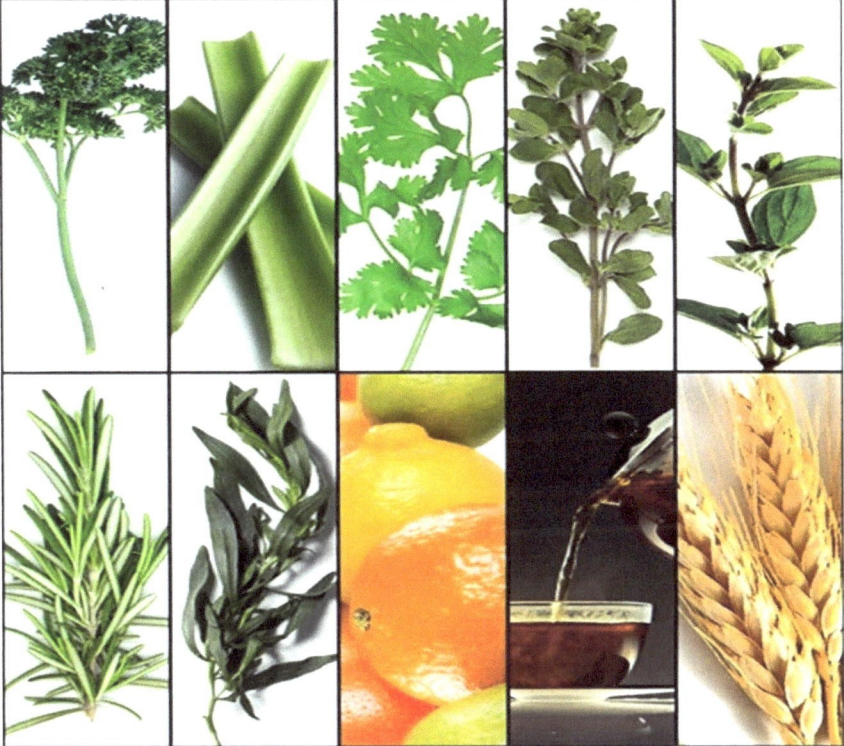

Figure 6-4 apigenin sources

Other than parsley, some of these herbs are not commonly uses. Bell peppers and garlic may be more accessible.

Flavonoids can be fun too! The cocoa bean is rich in flavonoids. I prefer the cocoa powder as my choice of these which I blend with unsweetened almond milk. If you add some walnuts and a few berries you have a flavonoid rich, nutritious drink. Dark chocolate is another acceptable source in moderation. Studies confirm that even once weekly intake of this class promoted better mental performance. They also reduce cardiovascular risk. They appear to have neuro-protective effects. Diabetics had improved blood vessel (endothelial function) when they drank a high cocoa flavanol drink. (part of this protection comes from epicatechin mentioned above)

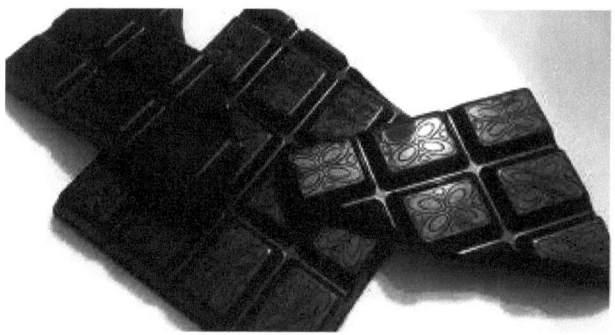

Figure 6-4 Dark chocolate as a flavonoid source

Bottom line, up your intake of flavonoids that are found in berries, cherries, currants, pomegranates, red and purple grapes, red onions, tomatoes, bell peppers, apple (skin), dark chocolate, and walnuts.

Catechin are Polyphenols is my second favorite phytonutrient. They are found in green tea, black tea, apples, avocados and berries.

Want to lose weight? Be sure to add catechins to your diet since they activate fat-burning genes in abdominal fat cells to assist with weight loss, and belly fat loss. According to research at Tufts University, catechins increase abdominal fat loss by 77 percent and double total weight loss.

Catechins showed many potentially health-promoting qualities: they are powerful antioxidants, support healthy gastrointestinal tract function, support detoxification function, and support repair of damaged DNA.

It has been shown to decrease the risk of many types of cancers. Research has shown a connection between catechin intake and a decreased cardiovascular disease. In addition to their other health-promoting activities, catechins have been found to be able to inhibit the oxidation of low-density-lipoproteins (LDL), the form of cholesterol that, when oxidized, is one of the contributing causes of atherosclerosis.

While drinking tea is a cultural ritual of community in Asia, it is now becoming a cultural ritual of wellness in the West. This is because green tea consumption has been shown to have many health benefits that researchers believe are related to the phytochemicals that it contains. Up your intake of green or black tea, apples, berries and avocado.

Catechin content of some foods

S.No	Food	Catechins, mg/serving	Catechins, mg/100g food
1.	Chocolate	23-30	46-61
2.	Beans	70-110	35-55
3.	Apricot	20-50	10-25
4.	Cherry	10-44	5-22
5.	Grape	6-35	3-17.5
6.	Peach	10-28	5-14
7.	Apple	20-86	10-43
8.	Red raspberry	2-48	2-48
9.	Strawberry	2-50	2-50
10.	Blackberry	9-11	9-11
11	Green tea	20-160	10-80
12.	Black tea	12-100	6-50
13	Red wine	8-30	8-30
14.	Cider	8	4

Hollman P, Katan M: Absorption, metabolism and health effects of dietary flavonoids in man. *Biomed Pharmacother 1997*

In one very large-scale study, the catechins in tea have been show to lower risk of stroke by approximately 20% when consumed in plentiful but still customary amounts. One cup of green or black tea in the morning, another in the afternoon, and a third in the evening were shown to provide the 30-50mg amount associated with risk reduction for stroke.

Phytochemicals in Vegetables - Glucosinolates

Just like our mothers told us, the foods we loved to hate as kids have turned out to be especially healthy for us. Members of the brassica family of vegetables, including broccoli, Brussels sprouts, cabbage, kale and bok choy appear to have significant cancer-preventive properties. Studies have shown that people who consume these vegetables frequently have a lower risk of developing a variety of cancers, including cancers of the colon, stomach and lung.

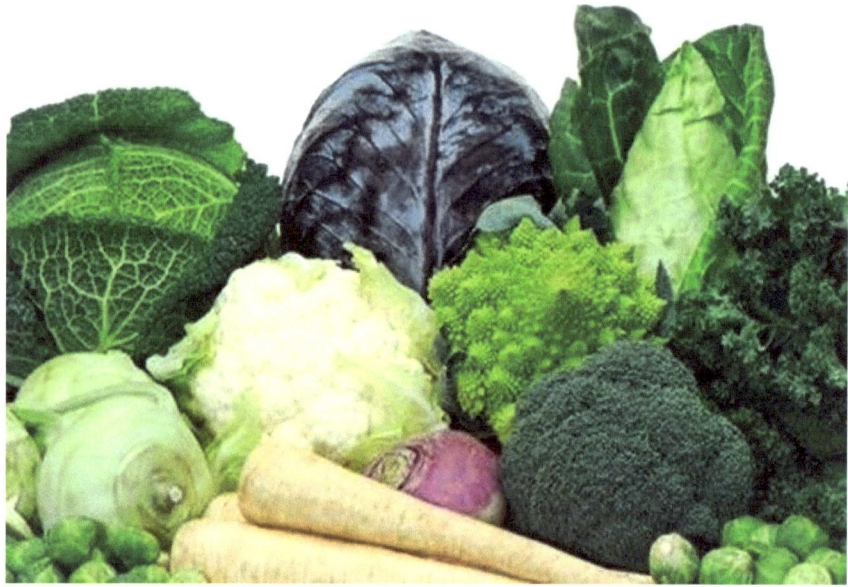

Figure 6-5 Glucosinolates sources

While these vegetables contain significant vitamin and mineral profiles, the key to their unique health-promoting abilities may be the presence of phytochemicals known as glucosinolates, members of the organosulfur chemical family.

Try to get some representation of each group as often as possible by choosing a wide variety of colors.

These phytochemicals seem to reduce the potential of carcinogens through their ability to beneficially modulate liver detoxification enzymes — they inhibit certain enzymes that normally activate carcinogens while also inducing other enzymes that help to dismantle active carcinogens.

One specific example of glucosinolate's effect on liver enzymes is the ability of one of the phytonutrients, indole-3-carbinol, to beneficially support the metabolism of estrogen. The liver metabolizes estrogen into either 16-alpha-hydroxyestrone or 2-hydroxyestrogen with the former suggested to promote cancer development and the latter suggested to oppose cancer development; the ratio of these two estrogen derivatives is used as a biomarker for the risk of developing hormone-dependent cancers such as those of the uterus and breast. Indole-3-carbinol promotes the conversion of estrogen to 2-hydroxyestrogen and decreases the amount of 16-alpha-hydroxyestrogen, a process that occurs in the liver. This promotion of 2-

hydroxyestrogen confers a decreased cancer risk. This nutrient is also available in the supplement DIM.

Carotenoids are another class of phytonutrients

Carotenoids include yellow, orange, and red pigment in fruits and vegetables. Dark, green, leafy vegetables are rich in the carotenoid, beta carotene, but the usual yellow color is masked by the chlorophyll, the green pigment in vegetables. The distinctive colors of mango, carrots, fall leaves, and yams are due to various forms of carotene, as is the yellow of butter and other animal fats. This pigment is important to our diet, as the human body breaks down each carotene molecule to produce two vitamin A molecules.

Not only do carotenoids help strengthen your eyesight, they protect against macular degeneration! They also boost your immunity to disease, they are powerful antioxidants that, in some studies, reduced the risk of cancer, heart disease and protected against the effects of aging.

Up your intake: Carotenoids are the yellow, orange, and red pigments found in foods like carrots, sweet potatoes, apricots, mangoes, pumpkin, tomatoes, papaya, peaches, and other similarly colored foods as well as dark green vegetables like broccoli and leafy greens

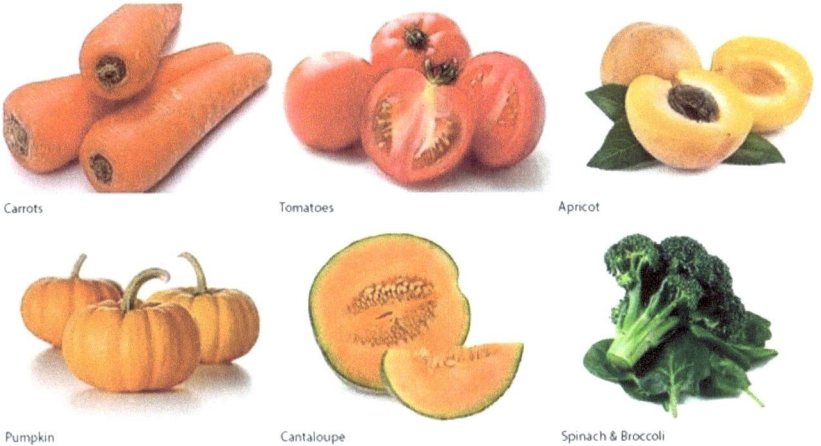

Carrots

Tomatoes

Apricot

Pumpkin

Cantaloupe

Spinach & Broccoli

Lycopene, canthaxanthin, and astaxanthin share a similar structure to carotene. The red tones of tomatoes, guava, red grapefruit, papaya, rosehips, and watermelon indicate the presence of lycopene.

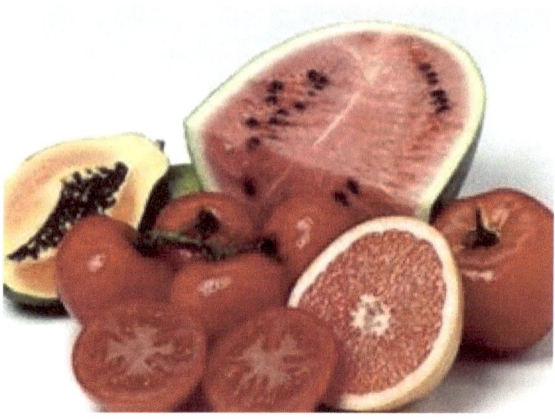

Figure 6-5 Lycopene source

In summary, most patients are deficient in the intake of fruits and vegetables to begin with. Try to get to the goal of at least 3 vegetable and 2 fruit servings per day. This alone, is still not optimal. If you limit yourself to your favorite fruit or vegetable, you will miss out on many of the miracle phytonutrients available that can have miraculous effects on preventing the damage of inflammation. They have been shown to go beyond that and provide many disease preventing properties.

Try to get at least 1 source of each phytonutrient in your diet. For anthocyanins focus in the red and purple fruit. For quercetin add in apples, red onions, teas, broccoli, and garlic. For Apigenin, add herbs like parsley, and other sources like garlic and bell peppers. For cocoa flavanols add dark chocolate! For catechins, berries, teas, chocolate, beans, and wine are sources. For glucosinolates, add green leafy vegetables like broccoli, bok choy, kale, and Brussel sprouts. For carotenoids, add in carrots, tomatoes, pumpkin and spinach. For lycopene add in red fruit like watermelon, red grapefruit, tomatoes, guava, and papaya.

Even easier, choose the rainbow of fruits. Try to get all the colors for each color is indicative of a specific nutrient class that is unique to that color. Eat red, purple, green, yellow, and orange fruit and vegetables on a frequent basis to get these health enhancing nutrients.

Chapter 9

EXERCISE

There are many entire books devoted to exercise. This book is not meant to be a work on exercise. Exercise, however is a critical part of health for a disease and death preventative measure. Exercise can reduce the incidence of morbidity and mortality and therefore has anti-aging properties

There are 3 main types of exercise, cardio, strength training, and flexibility. It is best to get a component of all 3 in your program. For many sedentary people, just initiating 1 of the 3 will move your body in the right direction. If you are only doing 1 of the 3, consider adding in a second routine.

Sittings Health Consequences

Americans are at higher risk for disease due to their high prevalence of sitting jobs. Sitting is very deleterious to your health. During sitting there is a lack of muscle contractions which reduces blood flow. The more you sit, the worse the health consequences. Every hour you sit decreases your life expectancy by 2 hours! Those who sit the most have a double risk of diabetes and heart disease. Prolonged sitting (6 hours uninterrupted) will counteract the positive effects of 1 hour of exercise! Those with the longest daily sitting where 8 years older biologically. Excessive sitting causes 3.8 % of all-cause deaths. It is truly lethal.

Ideally you should sit no more than 50 minutes if 1 hour. Sitting should be limited to 3 hours a day. Standing for 10 minutes is 1 way to avoid some of these consequences. In the next issue, another way to avoid the consequences of sitting.

Physical inactivity results in as many premature deaths as smoking! Adding exercise has been shown to reduce heart disease. You can reduce your risk if you do 30 minutes of moderate exercise 5 days a week or a total of 150 minutes a week. This can lead to a 14% risk reduction in premature deaths. This can be as simple as brisk walking. If you up the duration to 1 hour, then your risk reduction is improved to 20%. Most authorities recommend the 30 minutes or 150 minutes a week.

Weight training is often a neglected form of exercise. Some think weight training is only for muscle heads, but they are wrong from a general health standpoint, only about 23% of those over 45 get in adequate strength training.

Studies show you may be missing out on the most important aspect. Strength training reduced premature death by 23% and cancer by 31%! Longer life is just 1 aspect of the benefit.

Strength training benefits your cardiovascular system, decrease your risk for osteoporosis, improves mood, and self-esteem, sleep quality, and blood sugar control.

This is not to eliminate aerobic training which has positive benefits on brain function, cardiovascular fitness, endurance and stamina. Studies showing life prolongation are sparse and cancer protection absent.

In my opinion, a good balance of aerobic, strength training and flexibility is best.

For those confined to a desk job during the day, there is an easy solution to eliminating or reducing these consequences of sitting. It is called the nitric oxide dump. Here is how it works.

Nitric oxide is produced in your cell walls (endothelium) It promotes the health of your blood vessels and heart. Better blood supply fuels muscles and their development. You can increase your bodies productions with just 90 seconds of activity. This can be repeated 3-4 times daily for maximum effect. How it is done.

Squats- stand with feet hip width apart, toes forward. Move your butt back as in sitting while you balance with arms forward 10 times.

Alternating arm raises -alternate swinging your arms to 90 degrees angles 10 times.

Non-jumping jack- begin with arms down fist touching at pelvis, circle your arms over your head with fists touching 10 times.
Shoulder presses- Bring fists above your shoulders, elbows bent, then extend your arms straight overhead 10 times.
This can be done on lunch or brief breaks. Try it!

Exercise improves insulin sensitivity. It has been found to improve depression. Exercise reduces cortisol and stress, Exercise reduces appetite. Exercise triggers the release of BDNF (brain derived neurotrophic factor). This reduces atrophy and had the potential to reverse aging!

There is an "easier "method to streamline your exercise to the most effective and time efficient system. This is called high intensity interval training, or HIIT. HIIT is more effective than conventional cardio or weight training exercises and can be done in much less time.

How it works. For cardio, you warm up for 90 seconds on your exercise of choice, (stationary bike, elliptical, treadmill jogging, walking). Then, you put out maximum effort for 20-30 seconds, then repeat the cycle for 90 seconds. You want to complete at least 4 cycles. Caution for treadmill or jogging. These are higher risk exercises and ramping up should proceed cautiously, especially in new exercisers or older patients.

For weight training, instead of the traditional 3-5 sets on a muscle group, you will perform only 1 set. Here is how it is done. You will use lighter weight that you can lift easily about 8-12 times, BUT, you move the set infinitesimally slow. This is to avoid momentum and it will exercise the full muscle this way. Continue to the 8-12 goal repetitions, and until there is muscle failure for about 3 seconds. Then your set is complete. If you go beyond the 12 reps, then increase your weights next time.

HIIT is so intense that it should be done only a few times weekly at most. You can also do it with non-weight strengthening like pushups, dips, triceps rows, planks, etc.

There are many benefits to this form of exercise. You can be done in minutes and not hours! Attributed benefits include-Improved sleep, improved weight, improved immunity, improved bone density, improved mood, improved energy, improved athletic performance and improved libido.

It has also been shown to reduce inflammation, boost growth hormone production by 771%, improve bone density, relieve chronic pain and osteoarthritis and lower risk of cancer, heart disease, and diabetes by improving insulin sensitivity. WOW! What a list of benefits.

In conclusion, whether you choose aerobic training, weight training, flexibility exercise or HIIT, you will be rewarded with a healthier "younger body" with exercise. It is an essential to complete your process of reversing your bodies aging process.